50% OFF
Online CDN Prep Course!

Dear Customer,

Thank you for your purchase of this CDN Study Guide. Included with your purchase is **discounted access to our online CDN Prep Course**. Many CDN courses are needlessly expensive and don't deliver enough value. Our course provides the best CDN prep material, and with discounted access, **you only pay half price**.

We have structured our online course to perfectly complement your printed study guide. The CDN Prep Course contains **in-depth lessons** that cover all the most important topics, **600 practice questions** to ensure you feel prepared, and more than **450 digital flashcards**, so you can study while you're on the go.

Online CDN Prep Course

Topics Included:

- Concepts of Kidney Disease
- Hemodialysis
- Peritoneal Dialysis
- Transplant and Acute Therapies

Course Features:

- CDN Study Guide
    - Get content that complements our best-selling study guide.
- Full-Length Practice Tests
    - With 600 practice questions, you can test yourself again and again.
- Mobile Friendly
    - If you need to study on the go, the course is easily accessible from your mobile device.
- CDN Flashcards
    - Our course includes a flashcard mode with over 450 content cards to help you study.

To lock in your discounted access, visit mometrix.com/university/cdn or simply scan this QR code with your smartphone. At the checkout page, enter the discount code: **cdn50off**

If you have any questions or concerns, please contact us at support@mometrix.com.

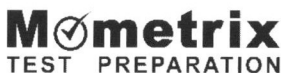

Certified Dialysis Nurse Exam
Practice Questions

CDN is a registered trademark of Nephrology Nursing Certification Commission, Inc., which is not affiliated with Mometrix Test Preparation and does not endorse this product.

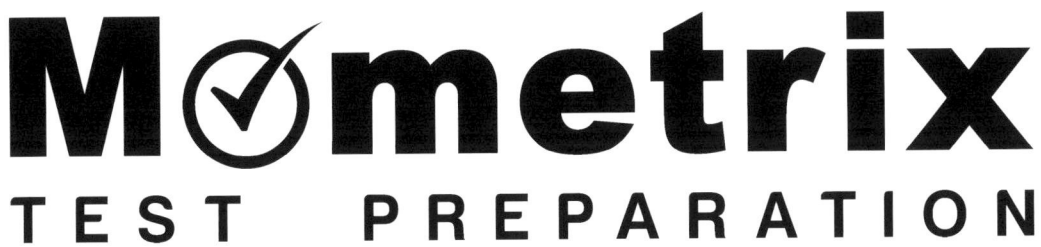

Dear Future Exam Success Story

First of all, **THANK YOU** for purchasing Mometrix study materials!

Second, congratulations! You are one of the few determined test-takers who are committed to doing whatever it takes to excel on your exam. **You have come to the right place.** We developed these practice tests with one goal in mind: to deliver you the best possible approximation of the questions you will see on test day.

Standardized testing is one of the biggest obstacles on your road to success, which only increases the importance of doing well in the high-pressure, high-stakes environment of test day. Your results on this test could have a significant impact on your future, and these practice tests will give you the repetitions you need to build your familiarity and confidence with the test content and format to help you achieve your full potential on test day.

Your success is our success

We would love to hear from you! If you would like to share the story of your exam success or if you have any questions or comments in regard to our products, please contact us at **800-673-8175** or **support@mometrix.com**.

Thanks again for your business and we wish you continued success!

Sincerely,
The Mometrix Test Preparation Team

Copyright © 2026 by Mometrix Media LLC. All rights reserved.
Written and edited by the Mometrix Exam Secrets Test Prep Team
Printed in the United States of America

TABLE OF CONTENTS

PRACTICE TEST #1 _____ 1

ANSWER KEY AND EXPLANATIONS FOR TEST #1 _____ 27

PRACTICE TEST #2 _____ 45

ANSWER KEY AND EXPLANATIONS FOR TEST #2 _____ 70

SHARE YOUR STORY! _____ 87

Practice Test #1

1. The primary advantage of using a Y-set with preattached double-bag system rather than a straight set for peritoneal dialysis is
   a. Ease of use
   b. Cost savings
   c. Decreased incidence of peritonitis
   d. Time saving

2. When a nurse is removing the needle from a buttonhole access on a patient who is HIV positive, a large volume of venous blood sprays into the nurse's mouth and eyes. Post-exposure prophylaxis (PEP) should include
   a. Basic 2-drug PEP
   b. Expanded 3-drug PEP
   c. Optional basic 2-drug PEP
   d. Observation and follow-up testing only

Refer to the following for questions 3-5:

   Rachel Stein is an 80-year-old woman with stage 3 chronic kidney disease.

3. When assessing an 80-year-old patient for kidney function, the nurse expects age-related changes to result in
   a. Decreased kidney size, decreased creatinine clearance, and increased BUN and serum creatinine
   b. Increased kidney size, increased creatinine clearance, and decreased BUN and serum creatinine
   c. Decreased kidney size, decreased creatinine clearance, and decreased BUN and serum creatinine
   d. Decreased kidney size, increased creatinine clearance, and increased BUN and serum creatinine

4. Stage 3 chronic kidney disease is characterized by
   a. eGFR 15–29 mL/min
   b. eGFR 30–59 mL/min
   c. eGFR 60–89 mL/min
   d. eGFR ≥90 mL/min

5. For elderly patients with chronic kidney disease who do not exhibit marked fluid overload, the need for dialysis may be delayed up to 1 year with
   a. Protein restriction and ketoacids
   b. Fluid and protein restrictions
   c. Protein restrictions and loop diuretics
   d. Fluid restriction and ketoacids

Refer to the following for questions 6-7:

> Anita Patel is a 46-year-old woman who undergoes CAPD following kidney failure associated with chronic glomerulonephritis.

6. Ms. Patel has developed a pericatheter mass. The most common method to differentiate a hernia from a hematoma or seroma is to
   a. Have the patient stand and bear down.
   b. Evaluate through auscultation and palpation.
   c. Examine with a CT scan.
   d. Examine with an ultrasound.

7. Once it is determined that Ms. Patel has a hernia, the patient is scheduled for CT with contrast. The patient has 2 L of dialysate containing 100 mL of contrast material (Omnipaque 300) instilled into the peritoneal cavity. After instillation, the patient should
   a. Immediately have the CT without any wait time.
   b. Walk about or remain active for 2 hours and then have the CT.
   c. Carry out normal routines for 5 hours and then have the CT.
   d. Lie in the supine position for 2 hours and then have the CT.

8. During hemodialysis, if blood is evident in the used dialysate, this probably indicates
   a. An incorrect pressure gradient
   b. Patient hemorrhage
   c. An incorrect dialysate formula
   d. A tear in the membrane

Refer to the following for questions 9-12:

> Grace Barry is a 46-year-old woman with end-stage kidney disease. Ms. Barry has had surgical creation of a polytetrafluoroethylene (PTFE) graft.

9. Following surgical creation of a PTFE graft, postoperative care should include
   a. Keeping the graft below the level of the heart
   b. Doing hand and arm exercises to promote maturation
   c. Elevating the extremity with the graft
   d. Checking blood pressure in the extremity with the graft

10. During hemodialysis, the nurse would expect Ms. Barry's temperature to rise by about
   a. 0.5 °C
   b. 1 °C
   c. 1.5 °C
   d. 2 °C

11. During routine hemodialysis, Ms. Barry's blood pressure should be monitored
   a. Every 15–30 minutes
   b. Every 30–60 minutes
   c. Every 60–90 minutes
   d. Before and after treatment

12. Ms. Barry has recently been diagnosed with bipolar disorder and is prescribed lithium. When should lithium be taken in relation to hemodialysis treatments?
    a. It should be taken prior to the treatment.
    b. It should be taken after the treatment.
    c. It should be taken only on days with no treatment.
    d. Timing is not an issue with lithium.

13. If all are available to a patient, the form of dialysis that provides the best control and the least inconvenience is generally
    a. In-center conventional daytime hemodialysis
    b. Home peritoneal dialysis
    c. Home hemodialysis
    d. In-center nocturnal hemodialysis

14. According to the Renal Physicians Association's clinical practice guidelines, to determine if dialysis should be avoided or stopped in patients with ESKD, one requirement is
    a. Family consensus
    b. Malignant disease
    c. Life expectancy <1 year
    d. Shared decision-making

15. The primary purification process of the dialysis water system is
    a. Deionization
    b. Filtering with activated carbon
    c. Reverse osmosis
    d. Addition of water softener

16. Which of the following medications is contraindicated to prevent muscle cramps during hemodialysis?
    a. Vitamin E
    b. Carnitine
    c. Quinine
    d. Oxazepam

17. If a patient on hemodialysis has a predialytic serum creatinine level that remains stable but a BUN level that is markedly increasing, the most likely cause is
    a. Change in residual urinary function
    b. Decreased dietary protein
    c. Incorrect dialysate
    d. Increased dietary protein

18. Endotoxemia associated with hemodialysis most often results from
    a. A break in aseptic technique
    b. Intestinal ischemia
    c. Contaminated dialysate
    d. A urinary tract infection

19. The number of milliliters of fluid transferred across a membrane per mmHg pressure gradient per hour is the
   a. Transmembrane pressure
   b. Osmotic ultrafiltration rate
   c. Extraction ratio
   d. Ultrafiltration coefficient

20. After a needle stick injury with exposure to hepatitis C–infected blood from a hemodialysis patient, post-exposure management includes
   a. Hepatitis C vaccination and ALT (alanine aminotransferase) test
   b. Immunoglobulin antiviral agent
   c. Immunomodulator
   d. Baseline testing for anti–hepatitis C virus and ALT test

Refer to the following for questions 21-22:

> Kim Wong is a 42-year-old patient who receives hemodialysis because of kidney failure caused by chronic glomerulonephritis. Recently, Ms. Wong has complained of increasing lethargy and itching and has exhibited slight jaundice. The physician suspects hepatitis C.

21. How frequently should patients on hemodialysis be tested for hepatitis C (HCV)?
   a. Monthly
   b. Every 3 months
   c. Every 6 months
   d. Every 6–12 months

22. If Ms. Wong tests positive for hepatitis C virus (HCV), which of the following interventions do the KDIGO guidelines recommend when providing hemodialysis treatments?
   a. Isolation of HCV-infected patients
   b. Adherence to strict infection-control procedures
   c. Use of dedicated dialysis machines for HCV-infected patients
   d. Discarding all dialyzers rather than reusing them

23. If a 24-hour urine quantitative protein test shows persistent proteinuria, this usually indicates
   a. Congenital abnormality
   b. Kidney infection
   c. Renal tumor
   d. Glomerular renal disease

24. An 80-year-old patient fell at home, fracturing her right hip. She was unable to move and lay on the floor for 24 hours before rescue. Routine medications include a β-blocker and statin. On admission to the hospital, the patient's urine is dark in color. The patient experiences generalized muscle weakness and pain. Laboratory tests indicate elevated creatine phosphokinase, serum myoglobin, and urinary myoglobin. Based on these findings, the patient is at risk of
    a. Pulmonary embolism
    b. Stroke
    c. Rhabdomyolysis
    d. Fat embolism syndrome

25. Which of the following factors may produce a false-negative finding in a urine dipstick for protein?
    a. Specific gravity of <1.01
    b. Specific gravity of >1.03
    c. Alkaline urine
    d. Presence of blood

26. The reason that hemodialysis requires a constant flow of fresh dialysate, rather than recycling the same dialysate, is to
    a. Reduce the risk of infection.
    b. Maintain a high pressure gradient.
    c. Maintain a low pressure gradient.
    d. Prevent clogging of the dialyzer.

27. At what point should a psychiatrist become involved in the care of a patient who is to begin dialysis for end-stage kidney disease?
    a. When the patient exhibits psychiatric/psychological symptoms
    b. At the onset of hemodialysis as part of the interdisciplinary team
    c. When the patient requests psychiatric care
    d. After the patient begins hemodialysis and emotional status can be assessed

28. If the vein downstream from an AV graft dilates over time, the best solution may be to
    a. Ignore the dilation.
    b. Move the AV graft.
    c. Surgically excise the dilated vessel.
    d. Convert the graft to an AV fistula.

29. The primary cause of neointimal hyperplasia of an AV graft is
    a. Blood turbulence downstream from the AV anastomosis
    b. Thrombosis at the site of the AV anastomosis
    c. Ischemia of the AV graft
    d. Allergic response to the graft material

Refer to the following for questions 30-32:

> Sadie Williams is a 52-year-old female with stage 4 chronic kidney disease resulting from hypertension and diabetes mellitus, type 1.

30. Ms. Williams complains of frequent nausea and a bad taste in her mouth. She states that her spouse reports that her breath increasingly has an "ammonia" or "urine" smell. The most likely cause is
   a. Dental caries
   b. Diabetic ketoacidosis
   c. Uremic fetor
   d. Gingivitis

31. Although Ms. Williams's control of her glucose levels had been poor, she reports that her glycemic control has improved in recent weeks, although she has had recent episodes of hypoglycemia. The most likely reason for this is
   a. Inadequate diet
   b. Hyperinsulinism
   c. Hypoinsulinism
   d. Diabetic ketoacidosis

32. Ms. Williams complains of increasing weakness and fatigue, resulting in difficulty in carrying out activities of daily living, such as cooking, cleaning, and even dressing; and this is causing her frustration and anxiety. The most valuable resource for this patient is likely a(n)
   a. Housekeeping service
   b. Physical therapist
   c. Psychiatrist
   d. Occupational therapist

33. Carbon filters in the water system are necessary to remove
   a. Organic materials and inorganic residue
   b. Electrolytes and endotoxins
   c. Microbial contamination
   d. Chlorine, chloramine, and organic materials

34. Sepsis that is associated with renal ischemia may result in
   a. Acute tubular necrosis
   b. Hydronephrosis
   c. Malignant hypertension
   d. Thrombosis

Refer to the following for questions 35-39:

Tony Pham is a 28-year-old male with a history of urinary tract infections. He comes to the ED with complaints of gross hematuria and bilateral flank pain.

35. An ultrasound is conducted to evaluate Mr. Pham's kidneys. Which of the following findings on ultrasound is diagnostic of autosomal dominant polycystic kidney disease?
   a. Two or more total cysts
   b. Two or more cysts in each kidney
   c. Four or more total cysts
   d. Four or more cysts in each kidney

36. Mr. Pham is most at risk for additional cysts in the
   a. Intestines
   b. Pancreas
   c. Spleen
   d. Liver

37. The gross hematuria associated with autosomal dominant polycystic kidney disease most often results from
   a. Rupture of a cyst into the renal pelvis
   b. Development of renal lithiasis
   c. A urinary tract infection
   d. An infected renal cyst

38. Mr. Pham reports that he has had three episodes of kidney stones over the previous 2 years. What type of kidney stone is most likely to occur in a patient with autosomal dominant polycystic kidney disease?
   a. Struvite
   b. Cystine
   c. Calcium oxalate
   d. Uric acid

39. If Mr. Pham develops sudden onset of excruciating pain in the lower back, right flank, and lower right abdomen, the most likely cause is
   a. Infection
   b. Ischemia
   c. Hepatic cysts
   d. Bleeding in a cyst

Refer to the following for questions 40-47:

> Tom Chang is a 65-year-old male patient with chronic kidney disease resulting from poorly controlled diabetes mellitus, type 2, and hypertension. Mr. Chang is aware that he will eventually need renal replacement therapy and is considering his options.

40. For a patient with chronic kidney disease, education about the different options for renal replacement therapy should generally begin at what GFR?

   a. ≤50 mL/min/1.73 m²
   b. ≤40 mL/min/1.73 m²
   c. ≤30 mL/min/1.73 m²
   d. ≤20 mL/min/1.73 m²

41. When teaching a patient about hemodialysis, the best way to determine that the teaching plan is geared to the patient's educational ability is to

   a. Routinely simplify instructions based on the patient's nonverbal cues.
   b. Assess the patient's abilities through a written test.
   c. Assess vocabulary level during conversations.
   d. Ask the patient directly about educational background and preferred style of learning.

42. When discussing options, the nurse points out that a disadvantage of hemodialysis as compared to peritoneal dialysis is

   a. Poor control of blood pressure
   b. Increased risk of hypertriglyceridemia
   c. Increased risk of malnutrition
   d. Increased incidence of back pain

43. If Mr. Chang chooses hemodialysis, which of the following would be a contraindication?

   a. Hemodynamic instability
   b. Metabolic acidosis
   c. Changes in mentation
   d. Hyperkalemia

44. When the nurse is teaching a patient about hemodialysis, the patient should understand that the primary advantage of short daily hemodialysis (at least 5-6 times weekly) is

   a. Improved serum albumin levels
   b. Better control of anemia
   c. Improved nutritional measures
   d. Reduced left ventricular hypertrophy

45. Mr. Chang is concerned about the time needed for dialysis. How many hours of peritoneal dialysis are approximately equivalent to 6-8 hours of hemodialysis?

   a. 12-20
   b. 20-36
   c. 36-48
   d. 48-56

46. Mr. Chang is considering CAPD. Which of the following may be a contraindication to CAPD?
   a. The patient has a history of cervical disk disease.
   b. The patient has a history of diverticulitis.
   c. The patient is legally blind.
   d. The patient is deaf.

47. Mr. Chang reports that his wife developed shingles, and he wonders if he should get the herpes zoster (shingles) vaccination. Patients with kidney disease considering the herpes zoster vaccination should be advised to
   a. Avoid the vaccination.
   b. Take 1 dose if age 60 or older.
   c. Take the dose if on immunosuppressive therapy.
   d. Take 3 doses if age 65 or older.

48. A 44-year-old man with a history of diabetes mellitus and hypertension is admitted to the hospital with increasing peripheral edema (2+ pitting), nausea and vomiting, lethargy, and generalized itching. The patient's blood pressure is 190/120 mmHg, pulse 86 beats per minute, respiration 26 breaths per minute. The patient's potassium (6.1 mmol/L) and phosphorus (10.2 mg/dL) are elevated, and BUN is 150 mg/dL and serum creatinine 14 mg/dL. Parathyroid hormone level is 885 pg/mL. Hemoglobin is 8.4 g/dL and hematocrit 27.2%. Glucose is 106 mg/dL. Based on these findings, the patient is most likely experiencing
   a. Liver failure
   b. Heart failure
   c. Rhabdomyolysis
   d. Uremia

49. During the diuretic phase of acute kidney injury, the patient should be closely monitored for dehydration, hyponatremia, and
   a. Hypokalemia
   b. Hypocalcemia
   c. Hypophosphatemia
   d. Hyperkalemia

50. Which part of the nephron resorbs urea, glucose, and amino acids?
   a. Proximal convoluted tubule
   b. Loop of Henle
   c. Glomerulus
   d. Bowman's capsule

Refer to the following for questions 51-55:

> Mary Ellen Locke is a 23-year-old female who developed acute kidney injury and renal failure after repeated bouts of glomerulonephritis. She has recently started peritoneal dialysis, APD with long-daytime dwell.

51. Ms. Locke calls to report that she has noted a small amount of blood in the effluent. The first question to ask the patient is

    a. "Do you have any abdominal pain?"
    b. "Do you feel weak or dizzy?"
    c. "Is there bleeding about the catheter exit site?"
    d. "Are you menstruating?"

52. Ms. Locke is very concerned about appearance and wants to know how much abdominal distention she should expect during dwell times. The average waist size increases by how much with CAPD?

    a. 1–2 inches
    b. 2–4 inches
    c. 4–6 inches
    d. 6–8 inches

53. Ms. Locke complains of a constant sweet taste in the mouth. The reason for this is probably

    a. Dental disease
    b. Development of diabetes mellitus
    c. Gastric reflux from increased abdominal pressure
    d. Absorption of glucose from dialysate

54. Ms. Locke has been losing weight and is becoming malnourished because her appetite is very poor and she feels full or slightly nauseated when she tries to eat a large meal. The best initial solution is probably to

    a. Eat immediately after draining the dialysate.
    b. Switch to APD.
    c. Take additional vitamin supplements.
    d. Eat small, frequent meals.

55. Ms. Locke's effluent shows many fibrin strands and clots, which are interfering with outflow. The recommended treatment is to

    a. Add heparin to the dialysate.
    b. Irrigate the tube with normal saline.
    c. Irrigate the tube with heparin.
    d. Provide exchange with amino-acid solution.

56. When the nurse is teaching a patient about peritoneal dialysis and dwell times, the patient should understand that the minimum dwell time necessary for adequate removal of waste products is usually about

    a. 1 hour
    b. 2 hours
    c. 3 hours
    d. 4 hours

57. Dialysate characterized as "ultrapure" should contain colony-forming units (CFUs)/mL of bacteria of
   a. <100
   b. <10
   c. <0.1
   d. <0.01

58. Which of the following may result in ischemic injury to the kidneys rather than nephrotoxic injury?
   a. Radiopaque contrast dye
   b. Amphetamines
   c. Anaphylaxis
   d. Tumor lysis syndrome

59. A patient has a Quinton catheter in place for hemodialysis while the AV fistula heals and matures. During hemodialysis, the red adaptor is used
   a. As the arterial port
   b. As the venous port
   c. As the arterial or venous port
   d. As a port for heparin

60. If a patient on CAPD has severe unremitting lower back pain, the best solution may be
   a. Changing to APD with no daytime dwell
   b. Changing to APD with daytime dwell
   c. A regimen of strengthening exercises for back and abdomen
   d. Remaining in supine position for an hour after completing a dwell

61. In medullary cystic disease complex type 1 (MCDC1), kidney failure usually occurs:
   a. In infancy
   b. Age 5-20
   c. Age 20-30
   d. After age 30

62. Which of the following is an example of a post-renal cause of acute kidney injury?
   a. Rhabdomyolysis
   b. Prostatic hypertrophy
   c. Acute glomerulonephritis
   d. Sepsis

63. When considering the stages of chronic kidney disease, a patient is considered in need of dialysis when the GFR falls to
   a. 60–89 mL/min/1.73 m^2
   b. 30–59 mL/min/1.73 m^2
   c. <15 mL/min/1.73 m^2
   d. <10 mL/min/1.73 m^2

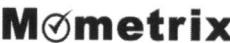

64. If a patient has been experiencing recent weight gain without generalized edema but with protuberant abdomen, and if the returns of dialysate are less than the instilled volume, the nurse should suspect

   a. Ultrafiltration failure
   b. Abdominal wall leak
   c. Overhydration
   d. Peritonitis

Refer to the following for questions 65-67:

   Following treatment for leukemia, Maria Santos, a 50-year-old woman, develops tumor lysis syndrome.

65. Which of the following responses to cell lysis may result in urinary obstruction and decreased glomerular filtration rates, leading to renal insufficiency and acute kidney failure?

   a. Hypermagnesemia
   b. Hypophosphatemia
   c. Hyperuricemia
   d. Hypercalcemia

66. Which electrolyte imbalances are likely to occur with tumor lysis syndrome?

   a. Hyperkalemia, hyperphosphatemia, and hypocalcemia
   b. Hypokalemia, hypophosphatemia, and hypercalcemia
   c. Hyperkalemia, hypophosphatemia, and hypocalcemia
   d. Hyperkalemia, hyperphosphatemia, and hypercalcemia

67. If Ms. Santos requires treatment for hyperuricemia, which of the following medications may be utilized to prevent uric acid crystallization?

   a. Loop diuretic
   b. Thiazide diuretic
   c. Alkalinizing agent
   d. Uricosuric agent

68. If post-dialysis blood values for BUN, sodium, and calcium are ordered, how soon after dialysis is discontinued should the blood be drawn?

   a. 20–120 seconds after discontinuation
   b. 2–5 minutes after discontinuation
   c. 5–10 minutes after discontinuation
   d. 15–30 minutes after discontinuation

Refer to the following for questions 69-75:

> James Woods is a 68-year-old man with end-stage kidney disease. He has been maintained on hemodialysis but has had to have repeated surgical procedures for vascular access and now wants to have a kidney transplant.

69. Mr. Woods is a candidate for kidney transplantation. The patient must register with the

   a. American Organ Transplant Association (AOTA)
   b. Organ Procurement and Transplantation Network (OPTN)
   c. United Network for Organ Sharing (UNOS)
   d. American Transplant Foundation (ATF)

70. When a patient such as Mr. Woods is on the waiting list for a kidney transplantation, what 3 factors are evaluated to determine if a match is appropriate?

   a. Blood type, HLA factors, and ages of donor and recipient
   b. Blood type, HLA factors, and race
   c. Blood type, HLA factors, and antigens
   d. Blood type, HLA factors, and antibodies

71. If Mr. Woods expresses concern that his insurance and available resources will not cover all of the cost of kidney transplantation, what Internet resource may provide the most valuable information?

   a. CMS (Medicare/Medicaid)
   b. UNOS Transplant Living
   c. National Kidney Foundation
   d. National Cancer Institute

72. Because Mr. Woods is concerned about the lengthy wait for a kidney, he is willing to consider a marginal kidney or a dual kidney transplantation. Which of the following would classify a cadaveric kidney donor as a marginal or expanded criteria donor (ECD) according to UNOS criteria?

   a. Age 55 at death
   b. Terminal creatinine of 1.3 mg/dL
   c. Previous history of slight cerebrovascular accident (CVA)
   d. Recent onset of hypertension

73. The primary purpose of dual kidney transplantation is to

   a. Provide more normal physiologic functioning.
   b. Increase success rates of marginal kidneys.
   c. Provide insurance in case one kidney fails.
   d. Prevent recurrent glomerular disease.

74. Which of the following is one of the critical major histocompatibility complex (MHC) genes for matching donor and recipient?

   a. HLA-C
   b. HLA-DQ
   c. HLA-DP
   d. HLA-DR

75. Following kidney transplantation, patients have increased risk of malignancies. The most common cancer that develops after transplantation is
   a. Renal cell carcinoma
   b. Lymphoma
   c. Skin cancer
   d. Liver cancer

76. Healthcare personnel caring for patients undergoing kidney transplantation should receive which of the following immunizations?
   a. Influenza (annual)
   b. Herpes zoster
   c. Hepatitis C
   d. DTaP

77. If a patient with a donor kidney develops sudden onset of hypertension 2 years after transplantation, the most likely cause is
   a. Vascular thrombosis
   b. Ureteral obstruction
   c. Graft rejection
   d. Arterial stenosis

Refer to the following for questions 78-79:

> A patient takes calcium carbonate 500 mg orally twice daily. Other medications include nifedipine extended-release (ER) 60 mg twice daily, aluminum hydroxide 600 mg 3 times daily, epoetin alfa 5000 units subcutaneously 3 times weekly, and iron polysaccharide complex 1 tablet daily.

78. Which of these medications should NOT be taken at the same time as calcium carbonate?
   a. Nifedipine ER
   b. Aluminum hydroxide
   c. Epoetin alfa
   d. Iron polysaccharide complex

79. Which of the patient's medications may increase risk of osteomalacia and refractory anemia?
   a. Nifedipine ER
   b. Aluminum hydroxide
   c. Epoetin alfa
   d. Iron polysaccharide complex

80. A hemodialysis patient's temperature per tympanic membrane thermometer is 37 °C. In order to reduce incidence of intradialytic hypotension related to inadequate vasoconstriction, the temperature of the dialysate solution should ideally be set at
   a. 37.5 °C
   b. 36.5 °C
   c. 38 °C
   d. 39 °C

81. The nurse is percussing the right kidney area of a patient using indirect fist percussion. The patient experiences pain when the nurse delivers a firm blow. This likely indicates
    a. A normal finding
    b. Renal cell cancer
    c. Congenital malformation of the kidney
    d. Infection or polycystic kidney disease

82. A 58-year-old female patient with type 2 diabetes and ESRD has developed numerous very painful firm brown nodules on both lower legs, with some of the nodules eroding and become necrotic. The skin color appears mottled, and the patient has decreased sensation. Based on these symptoms, the most likely intervention is
    a. Corticosteroids
    b. Immunosuppressive agents
    c. IV antibiotics
    d. IV sodium thiosulfate

83. A patient undergoing peritoneal dialysis and recovering from *Staphylococcus aureus* peritonitis is found to be a nasal carrier of *Staph*. The most commonly used prophylaxis is
    a. Rifampin 300 mg daily for 1 month
    b. Rifampin 300 mg twice daily for 5 days every 4 weeks
    c. Mupirocin cream intranasally once daily indefinitely
    d. Mupirocin cream intranasally twice daily for 5 days every 4 weeks

84. If there is an outbreak of *Aspergillus* infections in patients hospitalized with chronic kidney disease, an outbreak investigation should include review of
    a. Housekeeping procedures
    b. Handwashing procedures
    c. The water system
    d. Construction projects

85. During hemodialysis, a patient lying in supine position has chest pain, begins coughing, and shows evidence of cyanosis of distal extremities and lips. The nurse should suspect that the patient has
    a. Anaphylaxis
    b. A myocardial infarction
    c. Disequilibrium symptoms
    d. An air embolism

86. Following a renal biopsy, a compression bandage should be applied to the needle insertion site, and the patient should be positioned
    a. Supine and on bedrest for 24 hours
    b. On biopsy side for up to 60 minutes and on bedrest for 24 hours
    c. With no positional restrictions
    d. On biopsy side for 4 hours and on bedrest for 24 hours

87. Which water contaminant can cause ventricular fibrillation?
    a. Aluminum
    b. Chloramine
    c. Copper
    d. Fluoride

88. If a patient tests positive for a pericatheter leak, the most common treatment is
    a. Stopping peritoneal dialysis for up to 48 hours
    b. Surgical repairing of catheter site
    c. Removing peritoneal catheter and replacing at the same site
    d. Removing peritoneal catheter and using an alternate site

Refer to the following for questions 89-90:

> Ralph Jackson is a 27-year-old male diagnosed with anti-glomerular basement membrane disease (Goodpasture syndrome).

89. Goodpasture syndrome is typically characterized by kidney failure and
    a. Liver failure
    b. Pulmonary hemorrhage
    c. Pancreatitis
    d. Splenomegaly

90. The primary treatments for anti-glomerular basement membrane disease (Goodpasture syndrome) include
    a. Plasmapheresis and corticosteroids
    b. Blood transfusions and cyclosporine
    c. Plasmapheresis and IgG
    d. IgG and corticosteroids

91. The purpose of using a countercurrent flow, in which the blood flows in one direction and the dialysate in another, during hemodialysis, is to
    a. Aid osmosis.
    b. Aid diffusion.
    c. Decrease clotting.
    d. Remove larger molecules.

92. Which of the following organizations sponsors the "Save the Vein" campaign and supplies informational brochures for patients, as well as links to order "Save the Vein" wristbands?
    a. American Kidney Fund
    b. National Kidney Foundation
    c. American Nephrology Nurses Association
    d. National Organization for Renal Disease

93. According to the RIFLE (Risk, Injury, Failure, Loss, End-stage kidney disease) criteria, the stage of failure occurs with
    a. Serum creatinine increased by 1.5 times
    b. GFR increased by 25%
    c. GFR decreased by 50%
    d. Urine output <0.3 mL/kg/h for 24 hours

94. A patient with chronic kidney disease has anorexia but is steadily increasing in weight. The patient's potassium is 6.4 mEq/L, BUN 43 mg/dL, creatinine 3.6 mg/dL, hemoglobin 6.4 g/dL, and hematocrit 18.8%. Which of these laboratory findings has priority for intervention?
    a. Potassium
    b. Creatinine
    c. Hemoglobin
    d. BUN

95. The primary treatment for chronic kidney disease—mineral and bone disorder (CKD-MBD) is decreasing
    a. Hyperphosphatemia
    b. Hypercalcemia
    c. Hypernatremia
    d. Hyperkalemia

96. Which of the following is a risk factor for development of hernia in patients undergoing peritoneal dialysis?
    a. Small volumes of dialysate
    b. Supine position during dwell
    c. Anorexia and weight loss
    d. Obesity

Refer to the following for questions 97-106:

Madeline Stewart is a 64-year-old female receiving hemodialysis.

97. The renal dietitian has been working with Ms. Stewart to ensure the patient's diet meets physical needs. The best way to determine if the patient is in compliance and the diet is adequate is by
    a. Evaluating serum chemistries
    b. Reviewing the patient's food diary
    c. Asking the patient's family about diet
    d. Evaluating weight gain or loss

98. Ms. Stewart has recurrent iron deficiency, so she is on maintenance iron therapy. An appropriate iron treatment is
    a. 400 mg oral elemental iron daily
    b. 1000 mg IV iron monthly
    c. 200 mg oral elemental iron daily
    d. 50 mg IV iron weekly

99. When reviewing Ms. Stewart's food diary, which of the following sources of proteins should the nurse advise the patient is of low biological value?
    a. Eggs
    b. Tofu
    c. Dried beans
    d. Fish

100. Which of the following vitamins may be removed by hemodialysis?
   a. Vitamin A
   b. Vitamin B
   c. Vitamin D
   d. Vitamin K

101. How much additional protein should a patient on hemodialysis, such as Ms. Stewart, ingest every day in comparison to a healthy person?
   a. 10%
   b. 25%
   c. 50%
   d. 75%

102. What percentage of protein ingested by a patient on hemodialysis should be of high biological value?
   a. 30%
   b. 40%
   c. 50%
   d. 60%

103. What percentage of Ms. Stewart's diet should comprise carbohydrates?
   a. 20–30%
   b. 30–40%
   c. 40–50%
   d. 50–60%

104. How much fiber should Ms. Stewart include in her diet each day?
   a. 20–30 g/day
   b. 30–40 g/day
   c. 40–50 g/day
   d. 50–60 g/day

105. Which of the following foods is highest in insoluble fiber per serving?
   a. Apples
   b. Kidney beans
   c. Oatmeal
   d. Broccoli

106. Ms. Stewart is scheduled for intradialytic partial parenteral nutrition (PPN) to supplement her normal diet, as her serum albumin level is 2.9 and she has lost more than 10% of her normal body weight. The PPN is delivered per
   a. The venous port of the dialysis tubing
   b. The arterial port of the dialysis tubing
   c. A separate venous line on the opposite arm of the patient's fistula
   d. A separate venous line inserted between the arterial and venous needles

107. If a patient with acute kidney injury is prescribed sodium polystyrene sulfonate (Kayexalate), which of the following is a contraindication to administration of the drug?
    a. Diabetes mellitus
    b. Controlled hypertension
    c. Nausea
    d. Paralytic ileus

Refer to the following for questions 108-110:

> Susan Daly is a 37-year-old female who has chosen to begin hemodialysis after her kidneys failed as a result of systemic lupus erythematosus.

108. When evaluating Ms. Daly's upper extremity blood pressures preoperatively before formation of an AV fistula, a difference in blood pressure of 15 mmHg from one side to the other is graded as
    a. Normal
    b. Borderline
    c. Problematic
    d. Severe

109. The nurse is preparing written materials to help teach Ms. Daly and other hemodialysis patients about managing diet, medications, and other treatments. What is the most appropriate grade level for most patient materials?
    a. Second grade
    b. Fifth grade
    c. Seventh grade
    d. Ninth grade

110. When the nurse is teaching a patient about hemodialysis and all of the concepts that the patient must master, how many times should a concept be repeated before the patient is likely to have mastered the concept?
    a. 2–3 times
    b. 3–5 times
    c. 5–8 times
    d. 8–10 times

111. Following insertion of a peritoneal catheter and beginning of peritoneal dialysis, the nurse notes that the dressing over the site is damp. Which of the following tests should be done to help determine if the cause is pericatheter leak?
    a. Protein dipstick
    b. Glucose dipstick
    c. Hemoglobin dipstick
    d. Ketones dipstick

Refer to the following for questions 112-123:

> Janine Kim is a 30-year-old woman whose left kidney was removed at age 25. Now her right kidney is failing. Ms. Kim is preparing for hemodialysis and will have an AV fistula created.

112. According to KDOQI guidelines, the recommended first AV fistula should be which type?
   a. Femoro-saphenous
   b. Ulnobasilic
   c. Brachiocephalic
   d. Radiocephalic

113. When assessing veins and arteries prior to creation of a fistula, the minimum vein lumen generally needed for a successful fistula is
   a. 1.5 mm
   b. 2 mm
   c. 2.5 mm
   d. 3 mm

114. When evaluating Ms. Kim in preparation for creation of a fistula, the blood pressure difference between the arms should be less than
   a. 5 mmHg
   b. 10 mmHg
   c. 15 mmHg
   d. 20 mmHg

115. When conducting the Allen test to assess circulation of the radial and ulnar arteries, arterial insufficiency is indicated when the blanching persists for
   a. ≥2 seconds
   b. ≥3 seconds
   c. ≥4 seconds
   d. ≥5 seconds

116. For preoperative assessment of vessels, Doppler ultrasonography is often done under regional anesthesia of the arm because
   a. It is a painful procedure.
   b. Anesthesia causes the veins to dilate.
   c. Anesthesia causes the veins to constrict.
   d. The patient must hold completely still.

117. Following a period of maturation after the creation of an AV fistula, what diameter of the AV fistula is considered necessary before the fistula can be used for hemodialysis?
   a. 3 mm
   b. 6 mm
   c. 1 cm
   d. 1.5 cm

118. When auscultating Ms. Kim's AV fistula to listen for the bruit, the nurse notes that the bruit is very high-pitched. This may indicate
    a. Normal functioning
    b. Collateral circulation
    c. Stenosis
    d. Inadequate anastomosis

119. Ms. Kim asks about using the buttonhole technique for cannulation. When using the buttonhole technique for vascular access for hemodialysis, the needles are placed
    a. In the same sites in a graft
    b. In rotating sites in a graft
    c. In rotating sites in a fistula
    d. In the same sites in a fistula

120. When the nurse is teaching Ms. Kim about inserting a needle for hemodialysis, which of the following should the patient understand increases the risk of infiltration?
    a. Rotating the needle 180°
    b. Flushing the needle with NS after insertion
    c. Leveling the needle to the surface of the skin to advance
    d. Using a wet needle for insertion

121. Following formation of an AV fistula and the beginning of hemodialysis, the nurse notes that Ms. Kim's nail beds and skin on the hand below the fistula are cyanotic during hemodialysis, and the patient complains of pain in the hand. This is likely an indication of
    a. Steal syndrome
    b. Stenosis
    c. Aneurysm
    d. Infection

122. Ms. Kim is to have a trial cannulation of a newly matured AV fistula. The best time to carry out a trial cannulation is
    a. On a non-dialysis day
    b. On the first dialysis day of the week
    c. On the mid-week dialysis day
    d. On the last dialysis day of the week

123. The best way to determine if Ms. Kim needs glasses to adequately see the access site prior to beginning self-cannulation is to
    a. Refer the patient to an ophthalmologist for a comprehensive visual examination.
    b. Ask the patient if he or she routinely uses reading glasses for fine print.
    c. Observe the patient carefully during early cannulation attempts.
    d. Place a dot with ink on the patient's skin and ask the patient to touch it with a needle tip.

124. A patient on hemodialysis experiences persistent nausea during dialysis despite stable hemodynamics. The predialytic medication of choice to prevent nausea is
    a. Prochlorperazine
    b. Chlorpromazine
    c. Metoclopramide
    d. Ondansetron

Refer to the following for questions 125-133:

> James Brock is a 46-year-old man with acute kidney injury following an automobile accident that resulted in blood loss, abdominal injuries, and a fractured pelvis. Because his kidneys are not functioning adequately, the patient requires temporary hemodialysis.

125. Mr. Brock has a non-tunneled temporary hemodialysis catheter (NTHC) inserted into the femoral vein. Which of the following is a serious complication of femoral catheterization?
 a. Central venous stasis
 b. Pneumothorax
 c. Arrhythmia
 d. Retroperitoneal hemorrhage

126. In order to reduce the risk of complications, when an NTHC is inserted into the femoral vein, the practitioner should utilize
 a. Anatomic landmarks
 b. Angiography
 c. Real-time ultrasound
 d. Radiography

127. At the time of insertion of an NTHC into the femoral vein, what type of barrier precaution is advised for the patient?
 a. Head-to-toe sterile draping
 b. Face mask
 c. Standard access site sterile draping
 d. Standard access site sterile draping and face mask

128. The patient's NTHC should be replaced with a tunneled catheter if access for dialysis is needed for more than
 a. 24 hours
 b. 48 hours
 c. 5 days
 d. 7 days

129. For patients such as Mr. Brock with acute kidney injury, the treatment that has been shown to provide the best overall benefit is
 a. Furosemide
 b. IV normal saline
 c. Fenoldopam
 d. Nifedipine

130. Mr. Brock rings the bell frequently and often complains about staff members, insisting that they are neglectful and incompetent. The best response is,
 a. "I'm so sorry you experienced that. What can I do to help you?"
 b. "I'm sure that the other staff members are doing their best."
 c. "There are many other patients who need help too."
 d. "That is terrible. They should provide better care."

131. The patient is diagnosed with acute tubular necrosis and becomes increasingly depressed and withdrawn, stating that he wants to die rather than continue to suffer and to face the prospect of ongoing hemodialysis. The most appropriate response is to
    a. Reassure the patient that his condition will improve.
    b. Remind the patient that he is young and has much to live for.
    c. Provide the patient information about living with hemodialysis.
    d. Ask the physician for a psychiatric referral.

132. Mr. Brock has entered the oliguric phase of acute tubular necrosis when urinary output falls to
    a. <200 mL/day
    b. <300 mL/day
    c. <400 mL/day
    d. <500 mL/day

133. Mr. Brock becomes increasingly restless, irritable, and anxious, and has nausea, muscle cramps, and numbness and tingling of the fingertips and around the mouth. The ECG shows irregularities. The most likely cause is
    a. Hypokalemia
    b. Hyperkalemia
    c. Hyponatremia
    d. Hypernatremia

Refer to the following for questions 134-136:

> Joy Nguyen is a 58-year-old female with diabetes, type 2, and end-stage kidney disease. She has been treated with hemodialysis for 2 years.

134. Ms. Nguyen has developed numerous painful, firm, brown nodules on both lower legs, with some of the nodules eroding and becoming necrotic. Her skin color appears mottled, and she complains of decreased sensation. The most likely cause of these symptoms is
    a. Calcific uremic arteriolopathy (CUA)
    b. Peripheral arterial disease (PAD)
    c. Peripheral venous insufficiency
    d. *Staphylococcus aureus* infection

135. If Ms. Nguyen's ECG shows silent ST segment depression during hemodialysis, the most likely cause is
    a. Myocardial infarction
    b. Myocardial ischemia
    c. Coronary artery disease
    d. Left ventricular hypertrophy

136. Which of the following oral diabetic agents is acceptable for use in diabetic patients receiving hemodialysis?
    a. Tolbutamide
    b. Metformin
    c. Glipizide
    d. Exenatide

Refer to the following for questions 137-140:

> Ben Schwartz is a 58-year-old male who has been undergoing CAPD for the past year.

137. Mr. Schwartz informs the nurse that he has increased overall dwell time to compensate for skipping peritoneal dialysis 2 days per week. The best response is to
 a. Tell the patient to resume his previous schedule.
 b. Reassure the patient that this new schedule is appropriate.
 c. Recommend the patient switch to hemodialysis.
 d. Re-educate the patient about peritoneal dialysis.

138. Mr. Schwartz also reports that he had previously been doing 5 exchanges per day with CAPD, but now is doing only 2 per day but with much longer dwell times to compensate. The best information to provide the patient is that this practice
 a. Will result in reabsorption of effluent
 b. Is acceptable
 c. Will increase removal of toxins
 d. Will result in dehydration

139. Mr. Schwartz resumes his previous schedule for CAPD, but a month later he reports a change in his residual urinary output. Mr. Schwartz initially had approximately 400 mL of residual urine daily, but the volume has been decreasing. In response to this change in residual kidney function, the patient will most likely need
 a. No change in peritoneal dialysis
 b. Shorter dwell times or lower volumes of dialysate
 c. Longer dwell times or larger volumes of dialysate
 d. Dialysate with a lower concentration of glucose

140. Mr. Schwartz complains frequently about quality-of-life issues because of his need for dialysis. Which of the following assessment tools is most appropriate to assess quality of life?
 a. Katz index
 b. Mini-Cog
 c. Beck Inventory
 d. SF-36

Refer to the following for questions 141-143:

> Maureen Davis is a 70-year-old woman with diabetes mellitus, hypertension, and end-stage kidney disease. She is to have a catheter implanted for peritoneal dialysis and wants to try CAPD rather than hemodialysis.

141. How long prior to a patient beginning peritoneal dialysis should a catheter be implanted?
 a. 1 week
 b. 2 weeks
 c. 6 weeks
 d. 2 months

142. When teaching Ms. Davis about peritoneal dialysis, the nurse should advise the patient that one advantage to peritoneal dialysis over hemodialysis is
    a. Fewer restrictions in fluids and sodium
    b. Fewer treatments needed
    c. Less potential for complications
    d. Lower restriction on phosphorus intake

143. The nurse is concerned that Ms. Davis may not be a good candidate for CAPD. Which of the following is often a contraindication for peritoneal dialysis?
    a. Obesity
    b. Young adulthood
    c. Residual urinary function
    d. Cardiovascular disease

144. Treatment for nephrotic syndrome usually includes diuretics, lipid-lowering agents, and
    a. ACE inhibitors
    b. Beta-blockers
    c. Calcium channel blockers
    d. Vasodilators

145. If the dialysis center places HemaClips on dialysis tubing to prevent disconnection, what other precautions should be utilized?
    a. No other precautions required, as HemaClips are self-regulating
    b. Visible access sites/line connections and documentation of integrity every 30 minutes
    c. Visible access sites/line connections and documentation of integrity at the initiation and termination of treatment
    d. Visible access sites/line connections and monitoring by the patient

146. During the first dwell of peritoneal dialysis, a patient suddenly has severe shortness of breath. The immediate response should be to
    a. Sit the patient upright.
    b. Administer oxygen.
    c. Stop the dialysis.
    d. Advise the patient to take deep breaths and relax.

147. Following kidney transplantation, a patient develops a large lymphocele between the bladder and the transplanted kidney. The treatment of choice is usually
    a. Internal drainage into abdomen
    b. Sclerotherapy
    c. Instillation of fibrin glue
    d. Aspiration

148. For an end-stage kidney disease patient with difficulty sleeping because of restless legs syndrome, which of the following is generally considered the medication of choice?
    a. SSRI
    b. Benzodiazepine
    c. Dopamine precursor
    d. Steroids

149. In hemodialysis, *ultrafiltration* refers to
   a. Extraction of electrolytes
   b. Extraction of proteins
   c. Extraction of fluid
   d. Extraction of wastes/toxins

150. With hemodialysis, if the BUN is 100 at inlet and is 38 at outlet, the extraction ratio is
   a. 19%
   b. 38%
   c. 62%
   d. 79%

Answer Key and Explanations for Test #1

1. C: A Y-set with preattached double bag system, like the standard Y-set, also requires a flush-before-fill step, but the purpose is only to flush out air; bacteria are not likely to invade the system since there is no connection between the transfer set and the solution bag. This system is the most commonly used and is easier to use than other systems.

2. B: If a nurse's mucous membranes are exposed to a large volume of blood from a patient who is positive for HIV, post-exposure prophylaxis (PEP) should include the expanded 3-drug PEP because of increased risk of infection. If the volume were small, then the basic 2-drug PEP would be recommended. Nurses should be taught to use a 2-finger hold for removal of the needle from a buttonhole access because of the potential for blood spray.

3. A: The kidney becomes smaller in size and weight, and up to half of the glomeruli no longer function. Because of fewer functioning nephrons and decreased function in the loop of Henle and tubes, the creatinine clearance decreases and the BUN and serum creatinine increase. Urine is less concentrated because kidneys concentrate urine less efficiently.

4. B: Stage 3 is common in older adults with other disorders, such as cardiovascular disease, and in those at increased risk of cardiovascular events, such as myocardial infarction or stroke. At this stage, creatinine is usually within normal limits. Many patients will stabilize at stage 3, but some will progress to ESKD. Indications that kidney disease is progressing include decreasing eGFR, proteinuria, and hematuria.

5. A: For these patients, the need for dialysis may be delayed up to 1 year with protein restriction (very low–protein diet with 0.3–0.6 g/kg/day) and ketoacids as well as essential amino acids to compensate for the low-protein diet. Studies have shown that patients have no long-term adverse effects from this regimen. Patients must be monitored carefully to ensure adherence to the dietary restrictions.

6. D: Ultrasonography will show if the mass is fluid-filled. The ultrasound is relatively inexpensive and non-invasive. All different types of hernias (including ventral, pericatheter, umbilical, inguinal, and femoral hernia) are common with peritoneal dialysis, occurring in up to 20% of patients. Risk factors include use of high-volume dialysate, sitting, carrying out the Valsalva maneuver, obesity, and multiparity.

7. B: The patient should be advised to walk about or remain active for 2 hours because this helps move the dye about freely in the peritoneal cavity and into the hernia. The CT scan is not always necessary, depending on the site of the hernia. For example, the extent of an umbilical hernia may be quite evident on examination.

8. D: This probably indicates a tear in the membrane, allowing the blood to cross through the membrane and into the dialysate because the dialysate is lower in concentration. Blood leak detectors should sound an alarm if this occurs. Depending on the size of the tear, patients may rapidly lose blood, so the treatment must be stopped until the leak can be remedied.

9. C: Postoperative care should include elevating the extremity with the graft for several days after surgery to reduce edema. Exercises do not need to be done because the graft does not mature as an AV fistula does, but rather heals, so the graft can be used much earlier than an AV fistula, usually in about 2–3 weeks, after edema and erythema have subsided. The graft should be carefully assessed for pulse, bruit, and thrill.

10. A: Dialysis usually has little effect on the patient's temperature. Average temperature gain is usually about 0.5 °C. Elevations in temperature are most commonly caused by respiratory infections, urinary infections, and access site infections. Patients are at increased risk of infection because of impaired immune systems. Patients on dialysis may also develop fevers as part of a hypersensitivity response to medications or an allergic response to the dialysis circuit.

11. B: During routine hemodialysis, a patient's blood pressure should be monitored every 30–60 minutes, with increased frequency if the patient exhibits signs of hypotension (dizziness, weakness, pallor, faintness) or hypertension (facial flushing, headache). The blood pressure should be checked even when a patient is exhibiting no outward signs of blood pressure variation because patients may, for example, be dangerously hypotensive before they develop signs and symptoms. A drop in blood pressure may indicate that too much fluid has been removed and the patient's dry weight needs adjusting.

12. B: The lithium should be taken after each hemodialysis treatment because dialysis removes the lithium and the serum level will fall. Dosage and administration should be discussed with the patient's psychiatrist, and lithium levels should be checked frequently to ensure that lithium serum levels are therapeutic. Lithium has a narrow therapeutic range.

13. D: In-center nocturnal hemodialysis usually includes 3 nights of 7- to 9-hour treatments. This schedule increases the hours of dialysis and is done at a time the patient is sleeping so it does not interfere with daily activities. While home hemodialysis may be equally effective, the patient and partner must be trained, and the home requires modifications to accommodate a safe water supply and the equipment needed for dialysis.

14. D: Patients (and family) should be fully informed about the disease and should have advance planning. Forgoing dialysis may be considered for patients with poor prognosis or with marked risk factors. A process should be in place for conflict resolution in case of disagreement, and palliative services should be available.

15. C: Reverse osmosis removes up to 95% of contaminants and provides a protection against bacteria and endotoxins. While deionization may be used instead of reverse osmosis, it is more often utilized as a secondary treatment after reverse osmosis, but it does not remove bacteria or endotoxins from the water supply. Some deionizers exchange hydrogen ions for cations (calcium, sodium, aluminum), and some exchange hydroxyl ions for anions (fluoride, phosphate, chloride).

16. C: Quinine, which was once used routinely for treatment of muscle cramps, is effective as a treatment to prevent muscle cramps during hemodialysis, but it is no longer recommended because of multiple adverse effects, including thrombocytopenia, QT prolongation, and hypersensitivity reactions. Other medications that may help reduce cramping include carnitine supplements, oxazepam, and vitamin E. In some cases, increasing the sodium content of dialysate may reduce cramps, although care must be taken to avoid a sodium level so high that it increases thirst.

17. D: The most likely cause is increased dietary protein, so the nurse should review protein requirements with the patient and question the patient's diet. If both the serum creatinine and BUN level either increase or decrease similarly, then the nurse should suspect that a change has occurred in the patient's residual urine function or that the dialysis prescription needs modification.

18. B: Intestinal ischemia may occur if the blood pressure falls during a treatment session. In response to the ischemia, the cell walls of bacteria break down, releasing endotoxins that translocate per the intestinal barrier from the gut and may cause generalized inflammation as well as injury to the heart or other organs. In particular, the endotoxins cause peripheral vasodilation and impair the ability of the heart to contract adequately. In some cases, dialysis water may become contaminated with endotoxins.

19. D: The ultrafiltration coefficient depends on the permeability of the dialyzer membrane to water, varying according to the thickness of the membrane and the size of the pores. The ultrafiltration coefficient is designated as KUF. If, for example, the KUF is 10 and the transmembrane pressure is 100 mmHg, the patient would lose 1000 mL of fluid each hour.

20. D: Alanine aminotransferase (ALT) is a liver enzyme that increases with hepatitis C infection. Further testing may be done at 4–6 weeks and/or 4–6 months. There is no hepatitis C vaccination and no post-exposure prophylaxis, so those with exposure to hepatitis C should be monitored.

21. D: Patients on hemodialysis should be tested every 6–12 months for hepatitis C with the anti-HCV test, which is positive if a patient is infected. Hepatitis B, hepatitis C, and HIV are the bloodborne pathogens of most concern for hemodialysis patients. Hemodialysis patients have a higher prevalence of hepatitis C than the general population. According to KDIGO guidelines, if a new HCV infection occurs in a dialysis center and it is believed to be nosocomial, then all other patients should be tested.

22. B: According to KDIGO guidelines, if a patient treated in the dialysis center tests positive for hepatitis C virus, the best preventive method is adherence to strict infection-control procedures with all patients. Because HCV is a blood-borne pathogen, infection-control procedures should be adequate to prevent other patients from contracting the disease. KDIGO does not recommend isolating HCV-infected patients or using dedicated dialysis machines for them. Dialyzers can be reused as long as strict infection control procedures are adhered to.

23. D: Protein found in the urine is usually albumin. A 24-hour test should result in fewer than 150 mg of protein. Glomerular renal disease interferes with the kidneys' ability to filter toxins, so that some toxins that should be excreted are retained in the blood, and proteins and red blood cells that should be retained are excreted in the urine.

24. C: If an older adult fractures a hip and lies immobile for long periods of time, the patient may develop muscle trauma and rhabdomyolysis, which can lead to kidney failure because of the release of creatinine and myoglobin from the damaged tissue. Because the patient was immobile, the cell membrane is damaged, allowing sodium and water to fill muscle cells. Neutrophils enter the edematous tissue and cause an inflammatory response and nephrotoxicity. The typical triad of symptoms includes muscle weakness, muscle pain, and dark urine. The urine becomes red-brown in color from leakage of myoglobin from the muscle cells.

25. A: A specific gravity of less than 1.01 may produce a false-negative finding in a urine dipstick for protein because the urine is dilute. Other factors that may result in a false negative are urine that has a high sodium content, urine that is acidic, and the presence of non-albumin proteinuria because the dipsticks detect albumin. Other factors may also result in a false positive. These include the presence of blood or semen in the sample; urine that is alkaline; contamination of the sample with detergents, disinfectants, or radiocontrast agents; and a specific gravity of greater than 1.03.

26. B: With a high pressure gradient, diffusion occurs more effectively. If the same dialysate were to recirculate, it would become less and less efficient as it approached the concentration of the blood, because solutes would move less readily from the blood to the dialysate. In hemodialysis, the used dialysate is discarded down the drain.

27. B: All patients undergoing hemodialysis experience some degree of stress and anxiety when faced with changes in their health status and their lives, and they may be more receptive to assistance from a psychiatrist if the professional has always been a part of the team.

28. D: In some cases, an AV graft may be placed if a patient's veins distend poorly or are quite small and appear inadequate for formation of an AV fistula, but continued use of the graft often results in dilatation of the vein. This dilatation may make the vein suitable for subsequent transitioning to an AV fistula, which is the preferred access because of lower risk of infection and better patient outcomes.

29. A: The primary cause is blood turbulence in the vein downstream from the AV anastomosis. The risk of neointimal hyperplasia is greater with an AV graft than an AV fistula. As the hyperplasia develops, it can obstruct the vein, decreasing the blood flow in the graft and increasing bleeding when the needle is removed because of increased pressure within the graft. Over time, thrombosis of the graft may occur.

30. C: The most likely cause is uremic fetor, which develops as chronic kidney disease progresses to stage 5, kidney failure. As excess urea in the body breaks down in the saliva, it produces ammonia, which gives off a urine-like odor.

31. B: Hyperinsulinism is a common occurrence with kidney failure. The half-life of insulin is also prolonged, so patients are likely to require decreased doses of insulin (or in some cases, no insulin), and are at risk for hypoglycemia.

32. D: The occupational therapist can assess the patient in the home environment and can determine whether modifications or assistive devices could help the patient to manage better and to remain as independent as possible. If the patient's frustration and anxiety persist, the patient may benefit from a psychiatrist or other therapist.

33. D: Chlorine, chloramine, and organic materials are present in municipal water supplies and must be removed because they can degrade the reverse osmosis membranes. If this occurs, hemolysis can occur. Because these filters hold organic materials, they are at increased risk of bacterial contamination, so they should be replaced when exhausted, not reprocessed. Often, 2 carbon filters are used in series.

34. A: Acute tubular necrosis is the most common cause of acute kidney injury. The 3 primary causes of acute tubular necrosis are ischemia, sepsis, and nephrotoxins. Ischemia results in damage to the basement membrane and damage to the tubular epithelium, while nephrotoxins result in necrosis of the tubular epithelial cells, which in turn obstructs the tubules. This condition may be reversible if treated promptly.

35. A: The patient is presenting with typical signs and symptoms of autosomal dominant polycystic kidney disease—enlarged kidneys, gross hematuria, and flank (or abdominal) pain. Diagnosis is per ultrasound, and criteria varies according to age, reflecting the fact that the number of cysts tends to increase over time:

- Age <30: Two or more total cysts.
- Age 30–59: Two or more cysts in each kidney.
- Age ≥60: Four or more cysts in each kidney.

36. D: Hepatic cysts occur in up to one-half of patients with autosomal dominant polycystic kidney disease. Cysts may also occur in the pancreas and spleen, but they are less common. The cysts are distinct from the relatively harmless cysts that develop in the kidneys associated with older age.

37. A: The gross hematuria most often results from rupture of a cyst into the renal pelvis, especially as the cysts enlarge. However, in some cases, the hematuria may result from development of renal lithiasis or urinary tract infection. Bleeding usually recedes within a week of bedrest and adequate hydration. Persistent bleeding should arouse suspicion of renal cell carcinoma.

38. C: Calcium oxalate kidney stones occur in about 1 in 5 patients. Hydration of 2–3 L of fluid daily is encouraged to help prevent formation. Foods high in oxalate should be limited, including chocolate, soy products, nuts, nut butters, blackberries, blueberries, raspberries, figs, kiwis, Concord grapes, beans, beets, greens (collard, beet, kale, spinach, Swiss chard), squash, peppers, olives, and okra.

39. D: The most likely cause is bleeding in a cyst, causing it to rapidly expand in size. As cysts expand in size, the traumatized vessels stimulate angiogenesis, which in turn increases the risk of bleeding. If the bleeding is confined, the patient may not have hematuria. If the cyst ruptures, the patient may experience retroperitoneal bleeding and severe pain and/or hematuria.

40. C: Patients are often very stressed when dealing with the reality of dialysis, so they may be more receptive to education and better able to make a considered choice before their need for dialysis is imminent. Discussion should include different types of access (catheters, grafts, fistula) as well as different types of dialysis (CAPD, APD, home dialysis, nocturnal dialysis, in-center dialysis).

41. D: For example, a person with an advanced degree may be able to understand more complex explanations than a high school dropout, but this is not true for all people. When people are under stress, this can interfere with their ability to learn and to remember.

42. A: A disadvantage of hemodialysis compared to peritoneal dialysis is poor control of blood pressure, with the patient especially at risk for hypotension. Other disadvantages to hemodialysis include the need for heparin, which may increase the risk of bleeding; the need for vascular access; and the necessity of following a relatively strict diet. Peritoneal dialysis, on the other hand, increases the risk of obesity, peritonitis, hernia, malnutrition, hypertriglyceridemia, and back pain.

43. A: There are few contraindications to hemodialysis because it is used in life-threatening circumstances. However, hemodialysis is contraindicated if the patient exhibits hemodynamic instability or inability to coagulate blood, or if there is a lack of access to systemic circulation. Metabolic acidosis, changes in mentation, and hyperkalemia are all indications for hemodialysis. Other indications include fluid overload, elevated BUN (>90 mg/dL), elevated serum creatinine (≥9 mg/dL), drug toxicity, and signs of uremia. Hemodialysis is also indicated if there are contraindications to other forms of dialysis.

44. D: The primary advantage is reduced left ventricular hypertrophy, a common complication associated with chronic kidney disease and hemodialysis. Patients also experience improved physical functioning. These advantages hold true even if the total hours are similar to those of patients receiving hemodialysis in a center 3 times weekly for 4 hours. Short daily hemodialysis is usually done in-home rather than in a hemodialysis center.

45. C: With peritoneal dialysis, patients typically have 4 or 5 exchanges every 24 hours (often 3–4 during daytime hours and a longer one at night), with dwell times in the daytime typically averaging about 4–6 hours. Hemodialysis, on the other hand, is more commonly done for 3–4 hours 3 times weekly. Thus, hemodialysis is less time-consuming and requires less effort on the part of the patient, but the patient also may be more restricted in travel and less independent.

46. B: A history of diverticulitis is a contraindication to CAPD because the increased intra-abdominal pressure may result in rupture of the diverticulum. Other contraindications (not all absolute) include abdominal adhesions from previous surgeries, immunosuppressive drugs, colostomy, ileostomy, nephrostomy, or ileal conduit, and severe arthritis in the hands or impaired mobility of the hands. Inability to carry out the treatment independently is usually considered a contraindication. Patients who are legally blind or who have partial vision loss may be able to manage CAPD.

47. B: Such patients should be advised to take 1 dose if age 60 or older in order to decrease the risk of developing shingles and decrease the severity of shingles should they occur. However, post-transplant patients or any other patients receiving immunotherapy should not receive the immunization because the herpes zoster vaccine is a live virus vaccine, and those with depressed immune systems may develop the disease if they take the immunization.

48. D: The patient exhibits a number of signs and symptoms of uremia. Both diabetes and hypertension are risk factors, and increasing edema, nausea and vomiting, lethargy, and itching are common findings associated with uremia. The patient's blood pressure is uncontrolled on admission. The patient's laboratory results show signs of kidney failure, including hyperkalemia and hyperphosphatemia, as well as elevated BUN, serum creatinine, and parathyroid hormone. Additionally, the patient is anemic, with a low hemoglobin and hematocrit.

49. A: During this phase, the urinary output usually increases from about 1 L to 3–5 L per day because of osmotic diuresis. During the diuretic phase, the kidneys are able to excrete wastes but unable to concentrate urine, resulting in hypovolemia and hypotension. This phase may last for 1–3 weeks before the patient enters the recovery phase.

50. A: Glomerular filtration, in which fluids and solutes are filtered from the blood, is the first step in urine production, but reabsorption begins in the proximal convoluted tubule, which resorbs sodium, potassium, chloride, urea, glucose, and amino acids. Further reabsorption of electrolytes occurs in the loop of Henle, distal tubule, and collecting duct. The 3 processes involved in urine production are glomerular filtration, tubular reabsorption, and tubular secretion, which allows the body to reduce the concentration of substances in the blood, such as potassium or drugs.

51. D: While blood in the effluent is not generally a normal finding, it may occur for the first few initial treatments until the tissue is well healed. Blood may also be evident during menstruation, as the hypertonic fluid in dialysate can pull menstrual blood through the fallopian tubes and into the peritoneum.

52. A: Many patients are concerned about appearance when undergoing peritoneal dialysis and are worried about the kinds of clothing that they can wear. While there is some variation from one individual to another, the average waist size increases during treatment by only 1–2 inches. However, the catheter and any apparatus (tubing, bags) also take up space, so loose-fitting clothing is generally most appropriate. Some patients, especially those who are younger, may benefit from the assistance of a fashion consultant.

53. D: Some patients also develop a sweet aftertaste in their mouth after ingesting artificial sweeteners, such as aspartame. Patients may also complain of a metallic taste in their mouth, and this is often associated with the buildup of toxins in the blood between treatments.

54. D: Patients often feel full because of increased intra-abdominal pressure created with dwell and may feel nauseated if they try to force themselves to eat more. Simply adding vitamin supplements is not adequate, as patients need calories as well.

55. A: Treatment with heparin should be initiated when the fibrin strands are first observed because if obstruction occurs, irrigating with different solutions or with heparin is of little value. If the heparin is unsuccessful in improving outflow, then tPA (tissue plasminogen activator) instilled after normal saline irrigation is sometimes used to try to dissolve fibrin clots.

56. B: Most people use dwell times of 4–6 hours. Dwell times and the number of exchanges may vary depending on whether the patient is using CAPD, which requires no machine, or APD, which uses a machine to automatically cycle between dwell and drain, usually during the night.

57. C: Dialysate characterized as "ultrapure" should have CFU/mL of bacteria of less than 0.1 with endotoxin units (EU) of less than 0.03 EU/mL. Ultrapure dialysate may help to reduce inflammatory reactions in patients on long-term hemodialysis. Ultrapure dialysate is now recommended by some authorities for routine use, although current guidelines allow for product water that contains less than 100 CFU/mL and less than 0.25 EU/mL with maximum delivered dialysate levels of 100 CFU/mL and 0.5 EU/mL.

58. C: With ischemia, the inadequate perfusion results in impaired tubular endothelial function and damage to tubular cells, as well as cast formation. Other causes of ischemic injury include hemorrhage, volume depletion, prolonged hypotension, shock (cardiogenic, hypovolemic, and septic), and sepsis. Nephrotoxic causes of kidney injury include endogenous toxins from rhabdomyolysis and tumor lysis syndrome, antimicrobials, immunosuppressants, chemotherapeutics, illicit drugs (heroin, PCP, and amphetamines), and NSAIDs.

59. A: If a patient has a Quinton catheter (a non-tunneled central venous catheter) in place for hemodialysis while the AV fistula heals and matures, the red adaptor is used as the arterial port, and the blue as the venous port. The Quinton catheter, frequently used as a bridge device, has a dual lumen and is manufactured from soft pliable silicone. The Quinton catheter is available in different lengths to accommodate patients of different sizes.

60. A: Because of the increase in intra-abdominal pressure that occurs with a dwell, the center of gravity shifts, and this can put added stress on the lumbar vertebrae and muscles of the lower back. While bedrest and analgesia may provide some temporary relief, the pain is likely to recur unless the patient is in supine position during dwell time, but this is not practical with CAPD.

61. D: With medullary cystic disease complex type 1 (MCDC1) kidney failure usually occurs after age 30. Cysts form in the medulla of the kidney, resulting in asymmetric kidneys that are grossly scarred, interfering with the ability of the kidneys to concentrate urine. Symptoms include polyuria, metabolic acidosis, hyponatremia, hypertension, anemia, and progressive kidney failure.

62. B: A post-renal cause of acute kidney injury is an obstruction in the urinary tract below the kidney, such as in the ureter or the bladder neck, making the urine back up into the kidney. Prerenal causes of acute kidney injury are those conditions that decrease perfusion of the kidney before the arterial blood reaches the kidney. Intrarenal causes are those that produce injury through ischemia or toxins inside the kidney at the nephrons.

63. C: This is stage 5, and patients may also be considered for renal transplant if uremia is present. Some patients may live for many years with compromised kidney function, while others may progress quite rapidly to stage 5, depending on many factors, including the patient's general condition, adherence to treatment, and age.

64. B: The fluid builds up in the abdominal wall, resulting in weight gain, and the abdomen begins to distend, often asymmetrically (best viewed with the patient in standing position). The abdomen itself may appear edematous, with waistbands making a deep impression, for example.

65. C: If, following treatment for leukemia, a patient develops tumor lysis syndrome, cell lysis results in hyperuricemia, which in turn causes urinary obstruction because the increased levels of uric acid result in metabolic acidosis and crystallization of the uric acid in the kidneys. The kidneys are unable to adequately filter the crystals and the GFR decreases, resulting in renal insufficiency and acute kidney failure. Calcium and phosphorus ions bind and create calcium phosphate salts, which then precipitate in the renal tubules, increasing the risk of inflammation and obstruction.

66. A: The electrolyte imbalances that are likely to occur with tumor lysis syndrome are:

- Hyperkalemia: Intracellular potassium is rapidly expelled into the systemic circulation, resulting in muscular and cardiac abnormalities.
- Hyperphosphatemia: Intracellular phosphate is released, resulting in muscle cramping, tetany, cardiac dysrhythmias, and seizures.
- Hypocalcemia: Calcium levels fall as calcium and phosphorus bind, forming calcium phosphate, resulting in muscle cramping, tetany, cardiac dysrhythmias, and renal failure from acute nephrocalcinosis.

67. C: Commonly used medications include allopurinol, acetazolamide (Diamox), and sodium bicarbonate. Acetazolamide increases urinary pH by decreasing resorption of bicarbonate in the proximal tubules. Sodium bicarbonate alkalinizes the urine (target is 7) to increase the solubility of uric acid. Use of sodium bicarbonate must include careful monitoring of urinary pH.

68. A: Blood should be drawn within 20 seconds to 2 minutes after discontinuation of dialysis to obtain accurate results. Blood should not be drawn from fistulas or grafts, and it should be drawn from the opposite side as access in order to avoid trauma to the access site. Plasma levels of BUN increase up to 20% within 30 minutes, so timing of the blood draw is critical.

69. B: The Organ Procurement and Transplantation Network (OPTN is administered by the United Network for Organ Sharing (UNOS). The OPTN links all regional organ procurement organizations (OPOs) and transplant centers by a computer network. Patients may register with more than 1 center but may have to undergo medical evaluations at each center and will have to meet the centers' criteria.

70. D: The blood types must be compatible, although immunosuppression has allowed some success with ABO incompatibility. Human leukocyte antigen (HLA) factors must be evaluated because the more they match, the better the success rate. If blood type and HLA factors are suitable, then the donor's and recipient's blood samples are mixed to determine if the recipient produces antibodies against the donor.

71. B: This site provides detailed information about the entire process and has a section about financing a transplant, with links to various funding sources and guides for dealing with insurance and maintaining necessary records.

72. A: Age 55 at death (older than 50 years) would classify a cadaveric kidney donor as a marginal or expanded criteria donor (ECD) according to UNOS criteria. Other criteria include terminal creatinine of greater than 1.5 mg/dL, a history of diabetes mellitus, and a long history of hypertension. A donor is considered marginal if stroke is the cause of death. Another important consideration is the cold ischemia time (CIT). The longer the CIT, the bigger the risk of graft failure and mortality. Although no ideal CIT has been documented, extended CITs (longer than 36 hours) are of special concern.

73. B: The primary purpose of dual kidney transplantation is to increase the success rates of marginal kidneys, especially those from older donors. Studies indicate that success rates of double kidney transplantation are equal to or superior to rates for single kidney transplantation with marginal kidneys, especially after the first year. Double kidney transplantation is one way to expand opportunities for transplantation with marginal kidneys that might otherwise be discarded because of increased risk of failure.

74. D: HLA-DR, HLA-A, and HLA-B are the 3 critical major histocompatibility complex (MHC) genes for matching donor and recipient because these genes have the greatest effect on rejection of a donor organ. Other important but less critical genes are HLA-C, HLA-DQ, and HLA-DP. The human leukocyte antigen (HLA) genes are classified as class I (HLA-A, HLA-B, and HLA-C) and class II (HLA-DP, HLA-DQ, and HLA-DR). The greater the degree of matching between donor and recipient, the less likely the patient is to experience rejection of the donor organ.

75. C: Following kidney transplantation, kidney patients are at risk for numerous types of cancer, with up to 20% of patients developing cancer after 10 years. The most common cancer is skin cancer, usually non-melanoma, with squamous cell carcinoma being the most frequent. The next most common cancer is renal cell carcinoma, usually developing in native kidneys rather than transplanted kidneys. Renal cell carcinoma often occurs bilaterally and may be treated with nephrectomy, total or partial.

76. A: The CDC recommendations for healthcare personnel also include the hepatitis B series, varicella, and measles, mumps, and rubella (MMR) vaccines if not already immune, and a single dose of Tdap. Once an adult has received the Tdap vaccination, subsequent boosters should be with Td every 10 years. Family members and caregivers should also be advised to have the same immunizations in order to protect the patient.

77. D: The most likely cause is arterial stenosis, which can occur in up to 10% of patients within a few months or years after transplantation. Angiography is usually done to exclude other diagnoses and confirm stenosis. Treatment most commonly involves angioplasty and stent placement in order to ensure patency of the artery. Doppler ultrasonography may be used postoperatively to monitor progress and assess for hematoma formation.

78. D: Calcium carbonate can bind to iron polysaccharide complex and decrease the effectiveness of the iron, so they should not be given together. At least 2 hours should separate administration of the medications. Oral iron polysaccharide complex is given to patients with kidney failure to increase iron level because epoetin alfa cannot produce hemoglobin without adequate iron stores. Calcium is used to bind with phosphorus to decrease serum phosphorus levels and to compensate for a diet low in dairy products.

79. B: Aluminum hydroxide may increase the risk of osteomalacia and refractory anemia in a patient with chronic kidney disease and may also result in encephalopathy if aluminum toxicity occurs. Aluminum hydroxide is a phosphorus binder that prevents intestinal absorption of phosphorus, thereby decreasing serum phosphorus and increasing serum calcium. Because of the problems associated with toxicity, aluminum hydroxide is usually avoided and replaced with calcium binders. Aluminum hydroxide may interact with numerous other medications.

80. B: The temperature of the dialysate solution should ideally be set at 36.5 °C (0.5 °C below the patient's temperature). Dialysate that is too warm may result in vasodilation and reduced vascular resistance with resultant hypotension. Dialysate that is too cold may result in shivering and chills. In many centers, initial temperatures are set at 37 °C and then adjusted up or down, but this temperature may be too high for many patients.

81. D: This procedure should not elicit pain. Because the patient did experience pain, further tests, such as laboratory tests and imaging, are indicated to determine the cause. The nurse should also palpate the kidneys to determine if they are enlarged, although the left kidney is usually not palpable because of the position of the spleen.

82. D: The most likely cause of these symptoms is calcific uremic arteriolopathy (CUA), which is most often treated with IV sodium thiosulfate. Biopsies carry a high risk of mortality but may help to guide treatment; surgical debridement is contraindicated. Corticosteroids and immunosuppressive agents may worsen the condition. Some studies have indicated that patients on peritoneal dialysis seem to be at higher risk than those on hemodialysis, perhaps because phosphate levels tend to be higher with peritoneal dialysis. Secondary hyperparathyroidism is also an increased risk factor because of resultant hyperphosphatemia.

83. D: An alternative treatment is oral rifampin 300 mg twice daily for 5 days every 3 months. If patients who are nasal carriers are not treated for the nasal infection, they are at high risk for recurrent peritonitis. Repeated cultures should be done to ensure that the nasal infection is controlled.

84. D: An outbreak investigation should include review of construction projects in or near patient areas. *Aspergillus* spores are typically inhaled. *Aspergillus* infections are often associated with construction projects, which release the spores. These projects may even be outside of the facility, such as in an adjacent property, especially if windows are open or air filters become contaminated. Air-conditioning systems may also become contaminated, especially those placed in windows.

85. D: In supine recumbent position, the air often enters the heart (as opposed to the brain if the patient is sitting upright), generating foam in the right ventricle and into the lungs. If air returns from the lungs to the left atrium and ventricle, it can enter the arterial system and cause severe cardiac and neurological impairment.

86. B: The biopsy is usually done in the lower lobe of the kidney percutaneously and may be done with CT or ultrasound guidance. Following the biopsy, the patient should be assessed for hypotension, flank pain, increasing temperature, chills, dysuria, and bleeding.

87. D: Municipal water districts often add substances to the water supply to protect the health of the general public, but these substances may be harmful to patients on dialysis, so the dialysis system must filter out these substances. Fluoride, often added to prevent dental caries, can result in life-threatening ventricular fibrillation, as well as lesser complications, such as pruritus and nausea. Aluminum may cause bone disease and dialysis encephalopathy. Chloramine and copper may cause hemolytic anemia.

88. A: The most common treatment is to drain the abdomen and stop peritoneal dialysis for up to 48 hours because most leaks around the catheter will heal in a short period of time. If the leak persists, the patient may be placed on hemodialysis for a few days to allow more time for healing. If prolonged rest does not stop the leak, then the catheter may need to be removed and a catheter placed in another site.

89. B: Goodpasture syndrome, an autoimmune disorder that destroys collagen in glomeruli and alveoli, is typically characterized by kidney failure and pulmonary hemorrhage, although about 33% of patients may not exhibit pulmonary injury. Goodpasture syndrome is more common in males than females and is most common in males in their teens or 20s. Kidney failure may occur very rapidly. The disorder is often preceded by a viral infection or exposure to toxins, such as hydrocarbon solvents.

90. A: The primary treatments include plasmapheresis to remove the circulating antibodies and corticosteroids (or sometimes other drugs) to serve as immunosuppressive agents. Plasmapheresis is usually done daily for up to 14 days. Antihypertensives, such as ACE inhibitors and ARBs, are usually provided to control hypertension in order to protect the kidneys. Patients who require dialysis often have poor prognosis.

91. B: Dialyzers are less efficient if the flow is concurrent (both in the same direction). Diffusion occurs when two different fluids come in contact through a semipermeable membrane (such as the dialyzer membrane). The level of solute in the fluid is its concentration, and the difference in concentration between the blood (higher) and the dialysate (lower) causes the solutes to move from the higher concentration across the membrane and into the lower concentration.

92. C: The American Nephrology Nurses Association sponsors the "Save the Vein" campaign and supplies informational brochures (which can be downloaded) for patients, as well as links to order "Save the Vein" wristbands ("Save the veins—no IV/lab draws"). The purpose of the campaign is to educate both nurses and patients about the importance of meeting CMS goals of 66% of patients receiving an AV fistula, and KDOQI vascular access guidelines that stress the importance of protecting potential sites for fistulas.

93. D: According to the RIFLE (**R**isk, **I**njury, **F**ailure, **L**oss, **E**nd-stage kidney disease) criteria, the Failure stage occurs with urine output less than 0.3 mL/kg/h for 24 hours (oliguria) or anuria for 12 hours. Other indications include serum creatinine increased 3 times over normal, GFR decreased by 75%, or serum creatinine greater than 4 mg/dL with acute increase of at least 0.5 mg/dL. Loss is characterized by complete loss of kidney function for more than 4 weeks, and end-stage kidney disease is defined as complete loss of kidney function for more than 3 months.

94. A: Although the patient's laboratory results show multiple abnormalities, the priority for intervention is the elevated potassium because hyperkalemia puts the patient at risk for cardiac dysrhythmias and cardiac arrest, and the patient is nearing the critical value. Potassium values are categorized as follows:

- Normal values: 3.5–5.5 mEq/L
- Hypokalemia: <3.5 mEq/L; critical value: <2.5 mEq/L
- Hyperkalemia: >5.5 mEq/L; critical value: >6.5 mEq/L

95. A: Approaches include administration of phosphate binders, such as calcium acetate and calcium carbonate, and avoidance of the use of preparations with aluminum and magnesium. Secondary hyperparathyroidism should be treated with the activated form of vitamin D (because the kidneys can no longer activate it), using care to avoid hypercalcemia. Secondary hyperparathyroidism may also require cinacalcet, which mimics calcium.

96. D: Obesity is a risk factor because of the stress obesity places on the musculature. Other risk factors include sitting position during dwells and use of large volumes of dialysate. Patients who have undergone recent abdominal surgery are also at increased risk, as are multiparous women. Isometric exercises may strain the muscles and result in hernias. The Valsalva maneuver, which occurs when a patient coughs or strains to defecate, may also increase risk of hernia.

97. A: Patients may not always be accurate in a food diary or report of intake, especially if they know they are not following the prescribed diet. Also, in some cases, the diet may need to be adjusted according to laboratory findings.

98. D: An appropriate iron treatment is 50 mg IV weekly (25–100 mg recommended). Patients on hemodialysis should not receive oral iron because studies have shown that patients on hemodialysis do not benefit from oral iron, although it is beneficial for patients on peritoneal dialysis. Iron may be administered as repletion therapy only when iron levels fall, or as maintenance to prevent recurrence.

99. C: Protein sources are classified as being of high biological value (meaning the amino acids are in the balance required by the human body) or low biological value (meaning some amino acids are missing). Sources of protein of low biological value include dried beans and other plant-based proteins, such as whole grains, fruits, and vegetables. Sources of protein of high biological value include animal-based proteins, such as eggs, milk and other dairy products (cheese, yogurt), poultry, fish, and meat, as well as soy products, such as soy milk and tofu.

100. B: Water-soluble vitamins may be removed by hemodialysis. Water-soluble vitamins include the B vitamins and vitamin C. Fat-soluble vitamins are not removed by hemodialysis; these include vitamins A, D, E, and K. Patients should take supplements for water-soluble vitamins that are lost, including vitamin C (60–100 mg), folate (1–5 mg), vitamin B6 (2 mg), and vitamin B12 (3 mcg). Patients should be advised to discuss vitamins with their nephrologist and to avoid over-the-counter herbs and vitamins.

101. C: While patients with chronic kidney disease are usually on restricted protein, both peritoneal dialysis and hemodialysis result in loss of amino acids and proteins, with peritoneal dialysis causing loss of 5–15 g/treatment and hemodialysis causing loss of 10–12 g/treatment. Therefore, hemodialysis patients need to ingest about 50% more protein than a healthy person. Patients unable to maintain adequate protein intake are at increased risk of malnutrition and may require supplements or intradialytic parenteral nutrition.

102. C: At least 50% of protein ingested by a patient on hemodialysis should be of high biological value (i.e., complete proteins). Patients with chronic kidney disease are on restricted protein (0.7–0.8 g/kg/day) and often require supplemental amino acids. These patients should limit animal proteins (high biological value) because they are associated with more rapid progression of kidney disease. However, when the patients begin hemodialysis, the intake of protein must increase (1.2 g/kg/day) because protein is lost through hemodialysis, so patients should increase animal proteins.

103. D: For a patient on hemodialysis, approximately 50–60% of the diet should comprise carbohydrates (equal to about 1000 calories and 250 g of carbohydrates), although this percentage needs to include the glucose carbohydrates absorbed from dialysate (usually 300–400 calories). For patients with impaired glucose tolerance or increased triglyceride levels (reflective of carbohydrate intake), this percentage may need to be adjusted downward and compensated for with increased protein and fats.

104. A: A patient on hemodialysis should include 20–30 grams of fiber in the diet each day, as fiber helps to reduce lipid levels and gastrointestinal transit time. A diet high in fiber is believed to reduce the risk of cardiovascular disease. Fiber is generally classified as soluble (non-digestible and dissolves in water) or insoluble (non-digestible and doesn't dissolve), although a newer term is functional fiber, meaning non-digestible fiber with benefit to the body.

105. B: Fibers are polysaccharides that human enzymes are unable to digest. Beans, especially kidney beans, are higher across the board in insoluble fiber and total fiber than grains (oatmeal, pasta, bread, cereals), fruits (apples, bananas, berries, prunes, pears), or vegetables. Broccoli, for example, is quite low in both soluble fiber (1 g per serving) and insoluble fiber (0.5 g per serving). In the United States, insoluble fibers are given the caloric value of zero (0) per gram, while soluble fibers are given the caloric value of 4 per gram.

106. A: If a patient is scheduled for intradialytic partial parenteral nutrition (PPN) or total parenteral nutrition (TPN), the solution is delivered through the venous port of the dialysis tubing. It is usually initiated within 30 minutes of beginning dialysis and continues throughout the dialysis treatment. Some medications may be added to the parenteral nutrition solution, including insulin, heparin (to reduce adherence of microbes to the catheter lumen), and steroids (to reduce the risk of phlebitis).

107. D: Paralytic ileus is a contraindication because administration of the drug may result in necrosis of intestinal tissue. Sodium polystyrene sulfonate may be administered orally, or rectally as a retention enema. When the drug is in the bowel, potassium is exchanged for sodium; however, if hyperkalemia is severe, the patient may need dialysis to adequately decrease the potassium level.

108. B: A normal finding is a difference of less than 10 mmHg. All pulses (axillary, brachial, radial, ulnar) should be evaluated as well, and the Allen test should be carried out to help evaluate collateral circulation between the radial and ulnar arteries. Pulse oximetry may be used with the Allen test to improve reliability.

109. B: Even patients who are very well educated may have difficulty grasping medical information, especially if they are stressed or fatigued. The nurse should avoid the use of very long complex sentences or dense text, but should use highlighting, bulleting, and illustrations to help simplify information and make it more accessible.

110. C: Most people require that difficult concepts, such as health matters, be repeated 5–8 times before they are likely to have mastered them. To facilitate retention, the best practice is to vary the way the concept is presented, such as talking about it, providing reading material, reviewing it in a video or other electronic method, and using pictures/posters. Additionally, asking the patient to explain the concept or to provide a demonstration also increases retention and allows the nurse to evaluate the patient's knowledge.

111. B: If there is a pericatheter leak of dialysate, which is relatively high in glucose, the dipstick test should test strongly positive for glucose. The leak may be confirmed with contrast CT scan.

112. D: According to KDOQI guidelines, the recommended first AV fistula should be radiocephalic (above the wrist) because the fistula should be as distal as possible to allow replacement of the fistula should it fail. Vessels below a failed AV fistula are usually not suitable for access. The most common placement in the upper arm is brachiocephalic. Vessels need to be in good condition, and veins should be straight and able to accept a large-gauge needle.

113. C: The minimum vein lumen generally needed for a successful fistula is 2.5 mm, although smaller vessels down to 1.5 mm have been used successfully by skilled surgeons. The minimum size generally needed for the arterial diameter is 2 mm. However, size is only one important element, as the ability to dilate is also essential. Veins, for example, should demonstrate at least an internal diameter increase of 50% with the vein dilation test.

114. B: The blood pressure difference between the arms should be less than 10 mmHg. This is a normal finding. A difference of 10–20 mmHg is a borderline finding, and a difference of more than 20 mmHg is cause for concern. All upper extremity pulses should be assessed, as well as pulse oximetry. The Allen test should be carried out to assess circulation of the radial and ulnar arteries.

115. D: For the test, the patient should extend the arm and hand, palm upward. The nurse compresses both the radial and ulnar arteries at the wrist while the patient pumps the hand repeatedly to help the hand to blanch. Once the hand is blanched, the ulnar artery is released, and the duration of blanching of the palm is noted. Then, all compression is released and the procedure is repeated for the radial artery.

116. B: Anesthesia causes the veins to dilate, making them easier to visualize and assess. Doppler ultrasonography is used to measure the inner diameters of the arteries and veins as well as the flow velocity. However, central veins cannot be adequately visualized with Doppler ultrasonography. The vein dilation and arterial dilation tests are done during Doppler ultrasonography as well as vein mapping.

117. B: According to the "Rule of 6's," the diameter should be at least 6 mm and the depth below the skin less than 6 mm. Additionally, a straight segment of at least 6 cm should be present, and the AV fistula should accommodate a flow rate of at least 600 mL/min. This degree of maturation usually takes about 6 weeks but may extend up to 4 months in some patients.

118. C: The thrill should be low-pitched and constant. The other indications of stenosis include a pounding ("water-hammer") pulse, decreased thrill, intermittent bruit, edema of the access limb, increased venous pressure during treatment, recirculation, clotting of the extracorporeal system during treatment, excessive bleeding after removal of needles at completion of hemodialysis, "black blood syndrome," and decreased Kt/V and URR. Common sites for stenosis are inflow (juxta-anastomotic stenosis), outflow, and central vein.

119. D: The needles are placed in the same sites in a fistula, with one site for the arterial needle and one for the venous needle. KDOQI guidelines recommend teaching the patient to self-cannulate. The buttonhole technique cannot be utilized with a graft because the grafts lack muscle fibers to close the hole after the needle is removed. Using the same holes with a graft could result in a permanent opening and exsanguination.

120. A: When inserting a needle for hemodialysis, rotating the needle to any degree increases the risk of infiltration, and even one incidence of infiltration may damage an access. The nurse should be very gentle and proceed slowly when cannulating, and should level the needle to the surface of the skin before advancing it. Using a wet needle reduces the risk of infection and makes observing for flashback easier. The needle should be gently flushed with normal saline after insertion to ensure it is placed properly.

121. A: This is likely an indication of steal syndrome (i.e., dialysis access-related hand ischemia). The hand may feel noticeably cooler than the opposite hand. Steal syndrome may occur in up to 20% of accesses. Upper arm access increases the risk of steal syndrome, as do diabetes and peripheral arterial disease. Patients may complain of pain, paresthesia, and coldness of the hand during dialysis.

122. A: The best time to carry out a trial cannulation is on a non-dialysis day to avoid complications. If this is not possible, then the trial cannulation should be done at the mid-week dialysis day rather than the first day after a weekend without treatment, because there is less danger of fluid overload and electrolyte abnormalities. The selected needle size should be equal to or smaller than the vein without a tourniquet in place, usually size 17-gauge.

123. D: If the patient cannot do this accurately and without squinting, the patient may require reading glasses. A patient who wears bifocals may be able to see the site but may need to hold the head at an awkward angle to do so. In this case, the patient should obtain separate glasses to use during cannulation.

124. C: About 10% of patients on dialysis experience persistent nausea or vomiting, often related to hypotension or hypersensitivity reactions. If the nausea and vomiting are unrelated to hypotension, then metoclopramide 5–10 mg administered prior to dialysis may relieve symptoms. Some patients, especially those with diabetes, also develop gastroparesis, which may increase nausea and vomiting.

125. D: Other complications, common to all insertion sites, include hematoma, arterial puncture, and bloodstream infection. Bloodstream infection often causes the greatest risk. The use of both the internal jugular vein and the subclavian vein increase risk of air embolus and pneumothorax. Central venous stenosis and arrhythmias may also occur. Femoral catheterization should be the site of last resort and should be avoided if other sites are accessible.

126. C: In order to reduce the risk of complications, when a non-tunneled temporary hemodialysis catheter (NTHC) is inserted into the femoral vein (or any other vein), the practitioner should use real-time ultrasound. This is because vascular injuries—such as arterial punctures and hematomas—are fairly common if the practitioner uses only anatomic landmarks, which may be unreliable due to individual anatomic variation, especially in the position of the femoral artery and the femoral vein. While uncommon (about 0.5%), femoral catheterization may result in severe hemorrhage, so correct catheter placement is critical.

127. A: At the time of insertion of a non-tunneled temporary hemodialysis catheter (NTHC) into the femoral vein (or any vein), the barrier precaution advised for the patient is head-to-toe sterile draping. A chlorhexidine scrub (2%) is recommended for antisepsis, using a back-and-forth method of cleansing and allowing the solution to dry on the skin according to manufacturer's recommendations. The healthcare provider should use maximal barrier protection, including gown, mask, cap, and gloves.

128. C: The patient's non-tunneled temporary hemodialysis catheter (NTHC) should be replaced with a tunneled catheter if access for dialysis is needed for more than 5 days because of the increased risk of bloodstream infections with non-tunneled catheters. NTHCs may be left in place for up to 7 days with access sites in the internal jugular and subclavian veins. NTHCs should not be placed if dialysis access is expected for a period of longer than 3 weeks.

129. B: IV normal saline is administered to maintain a state of euvolemia or hypervolemia. Loop diuretics, such as furosemide, are frequently used to help maintain fluid balance but have not been shown to affect outcomes. Fenoldopam is sometimes used with hypertension to increase renal blood flow. Calcium channel blockers, such as nifedipine, are used as vasodilators/muscle relaxants, but their effectiveness is unclear.

130. A: It is important to acknowledge the patient's feelings without assigning blame to the patient or others, and to attempt to alleviate the problem. Simply spending extra time with the patient may help to allay the patient's anxiety.

131. D: Because the patient may, in fact, require ongoing hemodialysis if the condition becomes chronic, it is important to remain truthful, but the patient may need professional intervention to assess his depression and suicidal ideation.

132. C: The initial (onset) phase lasts for a few hours to a few days. It is followed in some patients by the oliguric or anuric phase, which lasts 10–16 days in oliguric patients. Some patients are nonoliguric; if this is the case, this phase lasts only 5–8 days. The third phase, the diuretic phase, lasts 7–14 days and includes a rise in GFR. The last stage is the recovery phase, which may take up to 2 years, although many patients never completely recover kidney function and about 5% require ongoing hemodialysis.

133. B: The most likely cause is hyperkalemia, a common finding with acute tubular necrosis, especially during the oliguric phase. Metabolic acidosis may also occur. The GFR decreases, resulting in increased BUN (azotemia), as well as hyperkalemia and other electrolyte imbalances, including hyperphosphatemia and hypocalcemia.

134. A: Calcific uremic arteriolopathy (CUA) is a life-threatening disorder associated with kidney failure in which arterioles become calcified, resulting in necrosis of the tissue. It is more common in patients with diabetic comorbidity, and incidence is higher in females than males.

135. B: Myocardial ischemia may be unrelated to coronary artery disease. Some patients may also exhibit increased levels of troponin T after dialysis, especially those prone to intradialytic hypotension. Troponin T is a marker for damage to the myocardium. Patients often develop myocardial ischemia as a result of intradialytic hypotension, which markedly increases the risk of cardiovascular-associated morbidity and mortality.

136. C: Glipizide, a second-generation sulfonylurea, is an oral diabetic agent that can be used for patients on hemodialysis and is generally the medication of choice. First-generation sulfonylureas (such as tolbutamide) should be avoided. Metformin (a biguanide) should also be avoided, as should the meglitinides (repaglinide and nateglinide). Glucagon-like peptide 1 analogs, such as exenatide, are contraindicated with hemodialysis. Most other oral diabetic agents require dose adjustments or should be avoided.

137. D: This patient does not understand some of the basic principles behind dialysis and needs re-education to ensure that he has a good understanding of the risks involved in skipping treatments. A fully informed patient is better able to make decisions. If the patient still wants to persist in having treatment-free days, then the patient may need to consider switching to hemodialysis.

138. A: While longer dwell times do often result in increased clearance of toxins, with excessive dwell times, a point of equilibrium is reached at which fluid and toxins no longer move, and some effluent may be reabsorbed back into the body as the osmotic gradient is lost. Patients should be advised to discuss any change in schedule of dwells with their nephrologist to ensure that the peritoneal dialysis is meeting the patient's needs and to prevent complications.

139. C: Residual kidney function is considered when prescribing peritoneal dialysate, but with a decreased urinary output, the patient's ultrafiltration rate to remove water must increase to compensate. The patient may also add additional exchanges or use dialysate with a higher concentration of glucose.

140. D: If a patient on CAPD complains frequently about quality-of-life issues (a common concern with patients on dialysis), the assessment tool that may be most appropriate is SF-36 (short-form health survey), which specifically assesses these issues. The method provides assessment in 8 areas: physical functioning, pain, role limitations associated with physical or emotional health, emotional status, social functioning, energy level, and general perceptions of personal health. This is a self-assessment tool that the patient can usually complete in less than 15 minutes.

141. B: At one time, even if a patient elected peritoneal dialysis, a backup AV fistula was created in case the peritoneal dialysis was not effective or the patient decided to switch to hemodialysis, but this is no longer recommended. Sometimes a peritoneal catheter is placed temporarily when a patient is going to have hemodialysis if the need for dialysis is urgent.

142. A: Fluid restriction is less stringent because of the more frequent dialysis, which removes excess fluid. Also, water passes through the peritoneal membrane more readily than through dialyzer membranes, increasing fluid loss. While hemodialysis patients must generally limit sodium intakes to 2–3 g daily, patients on peritoneal dialysis usually can have intake of 2–4 g daily.

143. A: Other contraindications include older adulthood and lack of social support, such as family members who can assist. Patients with ostomies or ventriculoperitoneal shunts are also usually advised against peritoneal dialysis. Indications for peritoneal dialysis include cardiovascular disease, younger age, adherence to treatment regimen, and adequate social support. The choice of peritoneal dialysis as opposed to hemodialysis should be made on an individual basis, considering many factors.

144. A: Treatment for nephrotic syndrome usually includes diuretics to reduce edema, lipid-lowering agents to decrease hyperlipidemia and slow atherosclerosis, and ACE inhibitors to reduce proteinuria. ARBs may also be used because they have similar protein-reducing effects. ACE inhibitors cause the efferent arterioles of the glomeruli to relax, reducing pressure within the glomeruli so that less protein is pushed into the urine. Commonly used ACE inhibitors for control of proteinuria include enalapril and captopril.

145. B: Other precautions include visible access sites and line connections and physical checking and documentation of integrity every 30 minutes. Patients should be educated about the importance of maintaining the visibility of connections at all times and of checking themselves. However, patients may fall asleep during treatments and should not be relied on for monitoring.

146. C: Because sudden onset of shortness of breath with the first dwell is consistent with hydrothorax, the immediate response should be to stop the dialysis to prevent further fluid from entering the pleural cavity. The patient should be assisted into sitting position and oxygen administered if necessary. Hydrothorax almost always occurs on the right side, so respirations should be evaluated. If necessary, a thoracentesis may be done to remove fluid. If the fluid withdrawn has high glucose content, this may help to confirm the diagnosis.

147. A: The treatment of choice is usually internal drainage into the abdomen, done laparoscopically. A lymphocele usually develops within the first year when lymphatic vessels leak lymph into the tissues. Patients typically complain of edema and pain and exhibit impairment of renal function. If the lymphocele is very small, sclerotherapy may be used, but the lymphocele may recur. Aspiration may increase risk of infection, especially if a drainage catheter is left in place. Fibrin glue is sometimes used.

148. C: A dopamine precursor, such as levodopa, is generally considered the medication of choice for restless legs syndrome (RLS), although benzodiazepines are also used. RLS is very common among patients with end-stage kidney disease. There is no objective test to diagnose RLS, so diagnosis depends on patient report of symptoms, which are typically an irritating sensation in the legs and feet that is relieved only by movement. RLS occurs during periods when the patient is at rest, usually prior to the patient's usual bedtime.

149. C: In hemodialysis, *ultrafiltration* refers to extraction of fluid from the vascular space. For ultrafiltration, the blood has a positive hydrostatic pressure, and the dialysate solution has a negative hydrostatic pressure. This difference in pressure pushes the fluid through a semipermeable membrane because fluid moves from an area of higher pressure to one of lower pressure. The difference between the positive and negative hydrostatic pressure represents the transmembrane pressure (expressed in mmHg).

150. C: The extraction ratio is the percentage of any solute, such as urea, that is removed across the dialyzer during hemodialysis. Formula:

$$\frac{\text{Inlet value} - \text{outlet value}}{\text{inlet}} = \text{extraction ratio (expressed as a percentage)}$$

$$\frac{100 - 38}{100} = \frac{62}{100} = 0.62 = 62\%$$

The extraction ratio is directly affected by the flow rate of blood through the dialyzer. The faster the flow of blood, the shorter period of time for extraction, so as the blood flow rate decreases, the extraction rate increases, and vice versa.

Practice Test #2

1. A new nurse in the critical care unit is unfamiliar with CRRT equipment being used and works very slowly because of the need to check procedures, which increases the workload of other staff members. The best solution is to
    a. Complain to the director.
    b. Advise the new nurse to take materials home to study.
    c. Allow the new nurse all the time needed to learn.
    d. Offer to assist and mentor the new nurse.

2. What is the purpose of the peritoneal equilibration test?
    a. Determine the amount of glucose absorbed from dialysate and the amount of urea and creatinine filtered into the dialysate in a 4-hour dwell.
    b. Determine the patient's serum urea and serum creatinine after a 4-hour dwell is drained.
    c. Determine the amount of urea in a 24-hour collection of drained dialysate compared to the amount of urea in the blood.
    d. Determine the amount of residual glucose that remains in the dialysate after a 4-hour dwell is drained.

3. Marked eosinophilia in a patient undergoing hemodialysis puts the patient at increased risk of
    a. Type A (anaphylactic) dialyzer reaction
    b. Type B (hypersensitivity) dialyzer reaction
    c. Hemolysis
    d. Air embolism

4. An adolescent patient has carried out peritoneal dialysis for 3 years, but on turning 18, the patient refuses further dialysis, stating he doesn't believe he needs it, although he is willing to take medications. He has moved out of his parents' home and into an apartment with three friends. The best response is to
    a. Refer the patient to a psychiatrist.
    b. Provide education and support to the patient.
    c. Advise the parents to get a court order mandating treatment.
    d. Advise the parents to cut off all support until the patient agrees to dialysis.

5. If the administration of a dialysis center bills for good and services that were not provided, it can be prosecuted under which of the following acts?
    a. Public Health Service Act
    b. Snyder Act
    c. Affordable Care Act
    d. False Claims Act

6. Peritoneal dialysate is rendered hyperosmolar with the addition of
    a. Glucose
    b. Sodium
    c. Bicarbonate
    d. Chloride

Refer to the following for questions 7-11:

> Sarah Novak is a 35-year-old woman who had a kidney transplant because of adult-onset polycystic kidney disease, but the kidney transplant failed, so she is again receiving hemodialysis while awaiting another kidney. Ms. Novak tends to develop hypotension during hemodialysis treatments.

7. Which of the following interventions may be indicated for a patient who develops hypotension during hemodialysis?

   a. Increasing the ultrafiltration rate near the end of the session
   b. Administering hypotonic sodium solution IV
   c. Utilizing sodium modeling
   d. Administering midodrine (Orvaten)

8. If Ms. Novak has a blood flow rate of 400 and the serum urea nitrogen is 100 at inflow and 35 at outflow, the urea reduction ratio (URR) expressed as a percentage is

   a. 35%
   b. 70%
   c. 50%
   d. 65%

9. The nurse has calculated the target weight loss for Ms. Novak's hemodialysis session, but the patient insists that the nurse has made an error and that the target is 1 kg too high. The nurse should

   a. Recalculate the target weight loss.
   b. Ignore the patient.
   c. Reassure the patient that the target is correct.
   d. Advise the patient that 1 kg is inconsequential.

10. Weight gain between hemodialysis treatments should not exceed

   a. 1% of dry weight
   b. 5% of dry weight
   c. 8% of dry weight
   d. 10% of dry weight

11. Ms. Novak asks the nurse what the chance is that the disease will pass to any children if her spouse is disease free. The nurse should advise the patient that a child will

   a. Have no risk of developing the disease
   b. Have a 25% risk of developing the disease
   c. Have a 50% risk of developing the disease
   d. Have a 100% risk of developing the disease

12. A patient with chronic kidney disease has started to make threats against a member of his family. He states that he wants the person dead and plans to use a gun to kill the person. The nurse's primary responsibility is to

   a. Refer the patient to a psychiatrist.
   b. Maintain the patient's confidentiality.
   c. Notify the police.
   d. Warn the person against whom the threats have been made.

13. In the formula for urea kinetic modeling (UKM), the K in the Kt/V formula stands for
   a. Duration of dialysis in minutes
   b. mL of fluid in the patient's body
   c. Dialysis flow rate
   d. Urea clearance (mL/min)

14. A hemodialysis center has set up a surveillance system to monitor bloodstream infections (BSIs). Once this event has been chosen for monitoring, what should be determined next?
   a. Methods of data collection
   b. Methods of data analysis
   c. Data elements for collection
   d. Time period for observation

15. For patients on oral iron, in order to increase absorption, patients should be advised to
   a. Take the supplement with dairy products, such as milk.
   b. Take enteric-coated preparations of the supplement.
   c. Take the supplement on an empty stomach.
   d. Take the supplement with phosphate binders.

16. During peritoneal dialysis, the concentration gradient of a substance, such as urea,
   a. Decreases
   b. Increases
   c. Remains consistent
   d. Varies widely

17. When a catheter is inserted for peritoneal dialysis, the length of the subcutaneous tunnel is usually
   a. 2–4 cm
   b. 4–6 cm
   c. 7–10 cm
   d. 10–15 cm

18. The physician has prescribed midodrine 10 mg for a patient to take 2 hours prior to hemodialysis. The most likely reason for this medication is to prevent intradialytic
   a. Hypotension
   b. Hypertension
   c. Muscle cramps
   d. Nausea and vomiting

19. A hospitalized patient who is incontinent of urine has undergone a renal scan. What precaution, if any, is needed by the nurse following the procedure?
   a. Gloves should be worn while handling urine and changing soiled linens.
   b. Gown, gloves, and facemask should be used when handling urine and changing soiled linens.
   c. No precautions are needed.
   d. A Foley catheter should be placed to safely collect urine.

20. **Glucose in dialysate must be heat-sterilized at a low pH in order to**
    a. Decrease generation of glucose degradation products.
    b. Increase generation of glucose degradation products.
    c. Prevent crystallization in the dialysate.
    d. Prevent the dialysate from becoming cloudy.

21. **Rigid non-cuffed catheters should be used for peritoneal dialysis for a maximum of**
    a. 24 hours
    b. 3 days
    c. 5 days
    d. 7 days

22. **With chronic kidney failure, vascular calcification results from**
    a. Hyperphosphatemia
    b. Hypophosphatemia
    c. Hypercalcemia
    d. Hyperkalemia

Refer to the following for questions 23-25:

> Salvador Rivera is a 68-year-old male with chronic kidney disease and diabetes mellitus, type 2.

23. **Mr. Rivera has severe peripheral nephropathy, hypertension, and proteinuria. His cholesterol level is 240. His GFR is 58 mL/min/1.73 m². Mr. Rivera has been taking metformin, an ACE inhibitor, a statin, and a thiazide diuretic. The patient's latest serum creatinine is 1.7. Which medication is cause for concern?**
    a. Statin
    b. ACE inhibitor
    c. Thiazide diuretic
    d. Metformin

24. **If Mr. Rivera's LDL level is 142, the goal of statin therapy and diet should be to decrease the patient's LDL to at most**
    a. <100 mg/dL
    b. <90 mg/dL
    c. <70 mg/dL
    d. <60 mg/dL

25. **Mr. Rivera is scheduled for a serum creatinine test. Mr. Rivera should be counseled to avoid which of the following for 8 hours before a serum creatinine test?**
    a. Strenuous exercise and red meat
    b. Dairy products
    c. A bath or shower
    d. Anticoagulant drugs

26. A patient is scheduled for an IVP. When the nurse is instructing the patient about preparation for the procedure, the patient should be advised to expect which of the following?
   a. There is no special preparation.
   b. The patient will be NPO for 8 hours prior to the test only.
   c. The patient will have a bowel prep and will be NPO for 8 hours prior to the test.
   d. The patient will have a bowel prep only before the test.

27. Diabetic nephropathy results from damage to the
   a. Glomeruli
   b. Renal artery
   c. Loops of Henle
   d. Proximal convoluted tubules

28. When a patient is severely dehydrated and hypotensive, the hypertonic plasma that results
   a. Stimulates the kidneys to secrete angiotensin
   b. Stimulates the parathyroid gland to release parathyroid hormone
   c. Stimulates the kidneys to release erythropoietin
   d. Stimulates the posterior pituitary to release ADH

29. If a patient with uremia passes urine that is foamy or bubbly, this probably represents
   a. Protein in the urine
   b. Rapid urination
   c. Phosphate crystals
   d. A normal urinary finding

30. As a leader of the interdisciplinary team, the nurse notes that a new team member is less productive than other team members and is often late finishing work. The best response is to
   a. Remind the entire team of their responsibilities.
   b. Speak directly with the team member about the observations.
   c. Report the team member to a supervisor.
   d. Give the team member a negative evaluation.

31. When utilizing Maslow's Hierarchy of Needs to set priorities in nursing care for hemodialysis patients, which level of needs has the highest priority?
   a. Safety and security
   b. Love and belonging
   c. Self-esteem
   d. Physiologic

32. An elderly patient undergoing hemodialysis has expressed the wish to die but has never requested a DNR order. During treatment, the patient experiences a cardiac arrest. The correct initial response is to
   a. Allow the patient to die.
   b. Carry out CPR and defibrillation.
   c. Carry out CPR only.
   d. Call the physician for guidance.

33. Backwashing to free residue from sediment filters in the water system should be done at least
    a. Every 8 hours
    b. One time daily
    c. Every 4 hours
    d. One time weekly

34. Standards that cover medical devices used for dialysis, such as dialyzers and blood tubing, are set by
    a. ESRD Network Organizations
    b. The Joint Commission
    c. FDA
    d. AAMI

35. A patient's urine osmolality is 300 Osm/kg. This probably indicates
    a. A normal value
    b. Dehydration
    c. Early kidney disease
    d. End-stage kidney disease

36. When a patient is being discharged from the hospital and will be referred to a home health agency for assistance with peritoneal dialysis, the best method to ensure that the patient understands the discharge plan is to
    a. Have the patient complete a post-discharge survey.
    b. Telephone the patient after discharge to discuss the discharge plan.
    c. Mail the patient a reminder of the discharge plan.
    d. Ask the home health agency for a follow-up report.

37. Which of the following symptoms is most specific for depression in a patient with uremia?
    a. Changing patterns of sleep with frequent insomnia
    b. Feeling tired and lethargic
    c. Repeatedly thinking about dying
    d. Exhibiting psychomotor agitation

38. The most common infection following kidney transplantation is
    a. Abdominal
    b. Pulmonary
    c. Urinary tract
    d. Cardiovascular

39. A patient at stage 4 kidney disease is considering options. The patient should understand that the best survival rate is associated with
    a. Post-dialytic transplantation
    b. Preemptive transplantation
    c. Hemodialysis
    d. Peritoneal dialysis

40. The hemodialysis center has instituted a "zero lift" policy. The primary purpose of such a policy is to
    a. Promote patient independence.
    b. Prevent injuries.
    c. Reduce liability.
    d. Reduce staffing.

Refer to the following for questions 41-47:

> Joseph Adler is a 38-year-old male with diabetes mellitus who has been on hemodialysis for the past 2 years. Mr. Adler's partner states that he has been increasingly withdrawn and disinterested, sleeping most of the day.

41. Mr. Adler is started on an SSRI (fluoxetine 20 mg daily) for treatment of depression. After 2 weeks, the patient reports no improvement. The patient should be advised that
    a. A different SSRI may be needed.
    b. SSRIs may be ineffective for the patient.
    c. Four to six weeks are needed to evaluate the response.
    d. The patient may respond better to other types of therapy.

42. If the patient continues to have persistent episodes of depression despite taking an SSRI for 3 months, which of the following non-pharmaceutical therapies may best help the patient to cope with the depression?
    a. Psychoanalysis
    b. Cognitive behavioral therapy
    c. Group therapy
    d. Electroconvulsive therapy

43. If one hemodialysis patient reacts to a complication with little apparent stress and copes well, and another patient, such as Mr. Adler, reacts to the same complication with severe stress and anxiety and copes poorly, the difference may lie in the patients'
    a. Sense of belonging
    b. Self-efficacy
    c. Resilience
    d. Hardiness

44. Mr. Adler has recently begun missing treatments and failing to take prescribed medications, despite the adverse physical response. When queried, the patient appears cheerful and insists that he is fine but "busy" and "forgot" about the treatments. The nurse should consider
    a. Suicidal ideation
    b. Dementia
    c. An electrolyte imbalance
    d. Anxiety

45. Mr. Adler states that one of his primary worries is that he is no longer able to work full-time but is not eligible for Medicaid. The patient is concerned that he cannot afford to pay for his insurance. The organization that may provide financial assistance is the

   a. American Association of Kidney Patients
   b. National Organization for Renal Disease
   c. National Kidney Foundation
   d. American Kidney Fund

46. When considering a hemodialysis patient's socioeconomic status, the three factors to focus on are

   a. Age, income, and education
   b. Residence, income, and race
   c. Income, education, and occupation
   d. Age, occupation, and income

47. Mr. Adler's depression seems to improve over time, although he continues to have multiple problems. Additionally, he brings a dog to a clinic appointment with him without explanation. If the staff is unsure if the dog is a service animal, a question that is legally permitted is

   a. "What kind of disability do you have that requires a service animal?"
   b. "Do you have proof that this animal is certified?"
   c. "What jobs has the dog been trained to perform for you?"
   d. "Can you ask the dog to demonstrate carrying out a task?"

48. The primary purpose of using an amino-based dialysate solution is for

   a. Increased ultrafiltration
   b. Decreased ultrafiltration
   c. Electrolyte imbalance
   d. Nutritional supplementation

Refer to the following for questions 49-50:

   Ramona Torres is a 50-year-old female who is admitted to the ED in acute distress. The patient reports having fever and dysuria for the past week.

49. Ms. Torres has developed sepsis as the result of a urinary tract infection, resulting in acute kidney injury (AKI) and the need for continuous venovenous hemofiltration (CVVH). The maximum dose for dialysis is

   a. 15 mL/kg/hr
   b. 25 mL/kg/hr
   c. 35 mL/kg/hr
   d. 45 mL/kg/hr

50. Ms. Torres has a catheter placed in the right jugular vein. In order to avoid puncture of the carotid artery when a venous catheter for acute hemodialysis is placed in the right internal jugular vein of a patient with sepsis, the best preventive is

   a. Anatomic landmark guidance
   b. Angiography
   c. Ultrasound
   d. Radiography

51. In order to slow the progression of chronic kidney disease in patients with chronic metabolic acidosis, sodium bicarbonate should be administered to maintain the serum bicarbonate level at
   a. 1.2 mmol/L
   b. 2.2 mmol/L
   c. 22 mmol/L
   d. 220 mmol/L

52. A patient who has been carrying out peritoneal dialysis for 3 years has recently been developing episodes of increasing dyspnea with treatment and is suspected of having a hydrothorax. The patient is to have radionuclide scanning with technetium. After the technetium is instilled into the peritoneal cavity, the patient should be advised to
   a. Lie quietly in the supine position between scans.
   b. Sit in a chair and lean forward.
   c. Remain ambulatory.
   d. Massage the abdomen.

53. Which of the following may result in a false positive for a urine albumin dipstick result?
   a. Increased urine sodium
   b. Specific gravity of less than 1.010
   c. Acidic urine
   d. Presence of blood

Refer to the following for questions 54-57:

> Josh Clark is a 40-year-old HIV-positive patient utilizing hemodialysis for end-stage kidney disease.

54. Mr. Clark often experiences intradialytic hypotension. Which of the following preventive measures is usually the best approach for patients who routinely experience intradialytic hypotension because of volume-related problems associated with large intradialytic weight gain?
   a. Increasing the patient's dry weight
   b. Extending weekly dialysis time
   c. Increasing restriction of fluid intake
   d. Increasing restriction of sodium intake

55. If Mr. Clark's predialytic serum total cholesterol level falls to <150 mg/dL, this probably represents
   a. An optimal cholesterol level
   b. Excessive statin dosage
   c. Poor nutritional status
   d. Incorrect dialysate

56. If Mr. Clark has persistent headaches during dialysis, the medication usually given to manage headaches is
   a. Aspirin
   b. NSAIDs
   c. Hydrocodone
   d. Acetaminophen

57. During Mr. Clark's hemodialysis session, a low-pressure alarm for venous pressure sounds. This could indicate
   a. Infiltration of the venous needle
   b. A clotted dialyzer
   c. Clotting in the access
   d. A poorly functioning central catheter

58. Prior to beginning treatment for diabetes, a patient's HbA1c was greater than 10%. What is a realistic target goal HbA1c for this patient?
   a. <9%
   b. <8%
   c. <7%
   d. <6%

59. A patient with kidney failure is to be assessed for possible vesicoureteral reflux (VUR). The test most indicated to confirm VUR is a(n)
   a. MRI
   b. IVP
   c. Voiding cystourethrogram
   d. Cystoscopy

60. In order to reuse dialyzers, the dialysis center must follow standards developed by the
   a. FDA
   b. CMS
   c. AAMI
   d. OSHA

61. Which of the following molecules has the highest molecular weight?
   a. Creatinine
   b. Urea
   c. Calcium
   d. Albumin

62. When needles are inserted into a PTFE graft for hemodialysis, how far apart should the needle tips be?
   a. At least 1.0 inch
   b. At least 1.5 inches
   c. At least 2.0 inches
   d. At least 2.5 inches

63. If a patient on hemodialysis exhibits a change in personality and demonstrates increasingly aggressive and threatening behavior, the best response is to
   a. Advise the patient that the behavior is inappropriate.
   b. Refer for psychiatric evaluation.
   c. Discontinue treating the patient.
   d. Enlist the help of family members.

64. According to the NHSN Dialysis Event Surveillance guide, the standardized infection ratio (SIR) is calculated based on the
    a. Number of bloodstream infections (BSIs) observed in a facility
    b. Number of observed BSIs divided by the number of at-risk patients
    c. Number of predicted BSIs divided by the number of observed BSIs
    d. Number of observed BSIs divided by the number of predicted BSIs

65. What color is arterial blood tubing for hemodialysis most often color-coded?
    a. Red
    b. Blue
    c. Green
    d. Yellow

66. If a patient with a Foley catheter requires a 24-hour urine collection for the creatinine clearance test, the proper procedure to collect the specimen is to
    a. Collect the urine from the catheter bag at the end of 24 hours.
    b. Place the catheter bag in a container of ice and collect urine every 8 hours.
    c. Place the catheter bag in a container of ice and collect urine every hour.
    d. Collect the urine from the catheter bag every hour.

Refer to the following for questions 67-71:

> Natasha Abramov is a 44-year-old patient who has received a deceased donor kidney because of polycystic kidney disease.

67. Since Ms. Abramov has received a deceased donor kidney, what information about the donor can be shared with the recipient?
    a. General location, age, and gender
    b. Age, gender, and race
    c. Address, name, and age
    d. Name, age, and gender

68. Which of the patient's drugs is classified as an antiproliferative and is often used in maintenance therapy after kidney transplantation?
    a. Cyclosporine
    b. Tacrolimus
    c. Prednisone
    d. Mycophenolate mofetil

69. Two weeks after kidney transplantation, Ms. Abramov has experienced an increase in temperature and flu-like symptoms, as well as weight gain of 2.5 kg in 48 hours, with decreased urinary output and pain in the operative site. The patient is scheduled for a core biopsy to determine if she is experiencing rejection. What guidance is usually used for the core biopsy?
    a. Anatomic guidelines
    b. CT scan
    c. Ultrasound
    d. Angiography

70. If the patient is confirmed through renal biopsy as having acute rejection, which of the following initial treatments is usually indicated?

   a. Corticosteroids
   b. OKT3
   c. High-dose cyclosporine
   d. High-dose tacrolimus

71. If Ms. Abramov develops hand tremors, back and abdominal pain, somnolence, loss of memory, and dark urine, as well as increased serum creatinine and BUN, the medication that is most likely responsible is

   a. Mycophenolate mofetil
   b. Cyclosporine
   c. Tacrolimus
   d. Prednisone

Refer to the following for questions 72-75:

> Stanley Mason is a 68-year-old man with end-stage kidney disease. He has decided against a kidney transplant and will begin hemodialysis.

72. When Mr. Mason begins hemodialysis treatments, he brings food with him to eat during his hemodialysis treatment. Patients should be advised to avoid eating during hemodialysis because ingestion of food may result in

   a. Hypotension
   b. Hypertension
   c. Nausea and vomiting
   d. Shivering and chills

73. During treatment, the nurse takes care to place the needles in antegrade position. The most important reason for placing hemodialysis needles in antegrade position is that

   a. It is easier to place the needles in this manner.
   b. It is less painful for the patients.
   c. It causes less scarring.
   d. It decreases the chance of infection.

74. Mr. Mason has weakness, and the nurse notes increasing muscle atrophy of the legs, decreased range of motion, and difficulty walking. The nurse should

   a. Advise the patient to be more active.
   b. Advise the patient to utilize a walker to prevent falls.
   c. Ask the patient to keep a record of activities.
   d. Ask the physician to refer the patient for physical therapy.

75. Mr. Mason has chronic itching and wants to try herbal or complementary treatment, as medications have provided little relief. The therapy that may be most beneficial is

   a. Acupuncture
   b. Aromatherapy
   c. St. John's wort
   d. Therapeutic touch

76. Long-term peritoneal dialysis places the patient at increased risk for which electrolyte imbalance?
   a. Hyperkalemia
   b. Hypokalemia
   c. Hypocalcemia
   d. Hypercalcemia

Refer to the following for questions 77-79:

   James Brown, a 70-year-old male with chronic kidney disease, presents in the ED with signs of uremia, including anorexia, nausea, fatigue, altered mental status, and signs of pericarditis with pericardial friction rub.

77. Immediate acute hemodialysis is needed to prevent
   a. Pulmonary emboli
   b. Atrial fibrillation
   c. Myocardial infarction
   d. Cardiac tamponade

78. Mr. Brown's blood urea nitrogen level is 130 mg/dL. What should the initial target urea reduction be?
   a. <20%
   b. <40%
   c. <60%
   d. <80%

79. When a venous catheter is inserted into the femoral vein for acute hemodialysis, the tip of the catheter should extend to the
   a. Inferior vena cava
   b. Superior vena cava
   c. Internal iliac vein
   d. Right atrium

Refer to the following for questions 80-87:

   MaryBeth Walker is a 28-year-old woman with a history of chronic glomerulonephritis affecting both kidneys. Because she is nearing end-stage kidney disease, she has decided to have hemodialysis treatments.

80. Ideally, for a patient with chronic kidney disease who will eventually have to have hemodialysis, a phlebotomist should draw blood from the
   a. Right antecubital area
   b. Left antecubital area
   c. Hand veins
   d. Foot veins

81. How many months prior to the expected onset of dialysis should a patient such as Ms. Walker have an AV fistula created?
    a. 1–2 months
    b. 2–4 months
    c. 4–6 months
    d. 6–9 months

82. Dialysis is usually considered in a patient with kidney disease when the patient's eGFR falls to about
    a. 5 mL/min/1.73 m^2
    b. 6.5 mL/min/1.73 m^2
    c. 8 mL/min/1.73 m^2
    d. 15 mL/min/1.73 m^2

83. If Ms. Walker's PTH level is high, the most appropriate referral is likely to a(n)
    a. Internist
    b. Nephrologist
    c. Endocrinologist
    d. Hematologist

84. Ms. Walker should avoid MRI with gadolinium contrast agent because it may result in
    a. Anaphylaxis
    b. Nephrogenic systemic fibrosis
    c. Glomerulonephritis
    d. Renal vascular stenosis

85. When the nurse teaches Ms. Walker about dietary restrictions, the patient should be advised to limit dietary phosphorus intake to
    a. 400–600 mg/day
    b. 600–800 mg/day
    c. 800–1000 mg/day
    d. 1000–1200 mg/day

86. According to KDOQI guidelines, patients with chronic kidney disease should restrict calcium intake to
    a. 1200 mg/day
    b. 1500 mg/day
    c. 1800 mg/day
    d. 2000 mg/day

87. In a patient with chronic kidney disease, such as Ms. Walker, metabolic acidosis results in
    a. Increased risk of cardiovascular disease
    b. Increased reabsorption of bone
    c. Increased risk of hemorrhage
    d. Increased risk of vascular calcification

88. During hemodialysis, how much blood is usually outside of a patient's body at one time?
    a. 50–100 mL
    b. 100–250 mL
    c. 250–400 mL
    d. 400–500 mL

89. A new occupational therapist has started working with the dialysis team, but this therapist has a different approach than the previous therapist, and some of the team members have begun complaining. As supervisor, the nurse's primary concern should be
    a. Ensuring that the team members are satisfied and working together well
    b. Informing the occupational therapist about needed changes in approach
    c. Assessing the quality of care the occupational therapist provides
    d. Establishing authority over the occupational therapist

90. If a patient has itching and stuffy nose that usually occurs only during hemodialysis, the most likely cause is
    a. Hypersensitivity reaction
    b. Hepatitis
    c. Scabies
    d. Anxiety

91. If the usual dose of potassium in dialysate is 2.0 mM, what is the usual dose for a patient who is taking digitalis?
    a. 1.0 mM
    b. 2.0 mM
    c. 3.0 mM
    d. 4.0 mM

92. A patient with chronic kidney disease who is on dialysis has been prescribed cinacalcet (Sensipar), probably indicating that the patient has
    a. Decreased parathyroid hormone
    b. Hyperkalemia
    c. Elevated parathyroid hormone
    d. Hypocalcemia

93. Which of the following infections is commonly associated with membranous nephropathy?
    a. Hepatitis A–related glomerulonephritis
    b. Hepatitis B–related glomerulonephritis
    c. Hepatitis C–related glomerulonephritis
    d. HIV-associated nephropathy

94. The most common reason for resistance to therapy with an erythropoiesis-stimulating agent (ESA) is
    a. Allergic response
    b. Hyperlipidemia
    c. Hyperparathyroidism
    d. Iron deficiency

95. Twelve months after receiving a kidney transplant, a patient experiences reduced urinary output and increasing serum creatinine levels. Ultrasonography shows hydronephrosis is present. The most likely cause is
   a. Renal artery stenosis
   b. Venous thrombosis
   c. Lymphocele
   d. Ureteral stenosis

96. The most important consideration for patients in their approaches to health beliefs and health practices is usually
   a. Educational background
   b. Cultural background
   c. Individual factors
   d. Socioeconomic status

97. When considering interdisciplinary communication, which of the following is an example of collegial communication?
   a. The nurse reports on the patient's condition in a team meeting.
   b. The nurse responds to a patient's questions about occupational therapy.
   c. The nurse chats about vacation plans with the physical therapist over lunch.
   d. The nurse provides one-on-one instruction to a patient regarding wound care.

98. The three processes involved in the production of urine are
   a. Glomerular filtration, hormonal stimulation, and tubular reabsorption
   b. Glomerular filtration, tubular reabsorption, and tubular secretion
   c. Glomerular filtration, ultrafiltration, and tubular reabsorption
   d. Glomerular filtration, sodium regulation, and tubular reabsorption

99. In which of the following groups are HIV-infected individuals most at risk for development of HIV-associated nephropathy (HIVAN)?
   a. Caucasian males
   b. African American males
   c. Asian females
   d. Caucasian females

Refer to the following for questions 100-102:

Carol Williamson is a 42-year-old female patient who presents with sudden onset of hematuria, fever of 39 °C, nausea, anorexia, severe left costovertebral angle pain, and tenderness in the left flank on palpation.

100. Based on these symptoms, the most likely diagnosis is
   a. Acute glomerulonephritis
   b. Chronic glomerulonephritis
   c. Acute pyelonephritis
   d. Chronic pyelonephritis

101. The physician orders a clean-catch urine sample for urinalysis and culture and sensitivities, a complete blood count, a dipstick leukocyte esterase test, and a nitrite production test. The purpose of the nitrite production test is to evaluate for the presence of
   a. Purulent material in the urine
   b. Bacteria in the urine
   c. Viral particles in the urine
   d. Fungi in the urine

102. Ms. Williamson is treated in the ED with a dose of parenteral ceftriaxone and is discharged with a prescription for ciprofloxacin 500 mg twice daily. How many days should the patient expect to take the oral antibiotics if no complications arise?
   a. 7 days
   b. 14 days
   c. 21 days
   d. 38 days

103. When influencing others to continuously improve practice, the nurse should recognize that the first step in the change process is to
   a. Believe in the possibility of change.
   b. Decide to bring about change.
   c. Take action to bring about change.
   d. Understand the results of change.

Refer to the following for questions 104-105:

> Denise Walker, a 62-year-old female on hemodialysis, complains of persistent itching during hemodialysis.

104. If Ms. Walker's itching persists and her Kt/V is 1.1, the first dialysis adjustment should be to
   a. Decrease Kt/V to <1.0.
   b. Increase Kt/V to >1.1.
   c. Increase Kt/V to >1.2.
   d. Increase Kt/V to >1.5.

105. If adjusting Ms. Walker's Kt/V and changing dialyzers does not relieve itching, the intervention most indicated is
   a. Gabapentin
   b. Moisturizers/oil bath
   c. Tacrolimus ointment
   d. UVB phototherapy

106. According to KDOQI guidelines, when administering hemodialysis to a patient, a facemask should be worn
   a. For all access connections
   b. If the nurse has a cough
   c. If the patient has a cough
   d. To discontinue the hemodialysis

Refer to the following for questions 107-112:

>Raul Rodriguez is a 52-year-old man with diabetes and end-stage kidney disease. Mr. Rodriguez uses CAPD but reports that his peritoneal fluid has become cloudy.

107. Which of the following medications may result in cloudy peritoneal fluid for patients on peritoneal dialysis?

   a. Calcium carbonate
   b. Beta-blockers
   c. ACE inhibitors
   d. Calcium channel blockers

108. Which of the following places a patient on peritoneal dialysis at high risk for peritonitis?

   a. Spiking of dialysis bags
   b. "Flush before fill" procedure
   c. Double-cuffed catheter
   d. Downward-directed skin exit site

109. Mr. Rodriguez's peritoneal catheter cultures positive for fungal organisms, indicating that the tube is colonized. The most likely intervention is

   a. Antifungal instillations
   b. Removal of catheter and temporary hemodialysis
   c. Replacement of catheter
   d. Oral nystatin until culture is clear

110. When patients are undergoing peritoneal dialysis, the most common pathway of infection resulting in peritonitis is

   a. Periluminal
   b. Hematogenous
   c. Intraluminal
   d. Transvaginal

111. If Mr. Rodriguez's CAPD requires a sample of peritoneal solution for evaluation of the cell count, the correct method of obtaining the specimen is to

   a. Aspirate directly from the peritoneal catheter.
   b. Invert the drainage bag a few times to mix the solution and aspirate from the bag port.
   c. Aspirate from the bag port without mixing the solution.
   d. Infuse 1 L of solution and then drain immediately and obtain sample from effluent.

112. If a sample of peritoneal fluid cannot be immediately processed, the inoculated culture bottles should ideally be stored at

   a. 35 °C
   b. 35.5 °C
   c. 37 °C
   d. 38 °C

113. Patients undergoing home nocturnal hemodialysis are required to have which item within arm's reach while undergoing dialysis?
   a. Tourniquet
   b. Kelly clamp
   c. Whistle
   d. Telephone

Refer to the following for questions 114-118:

> Grace Johnson is a 58-year-old female with diabetes mellitus, type 1, who is undergoing hemodialysis. The patient has had problems tolerating hemodialysis, with numerous complications.

114. Ms. Johnson complains of severe muscle pain and stiffness. Medications include calcitriol 0.25 mg daily, atorvastatin 20 mg daily, insulin glargine 26 units twice daily, regular insulin per sliding scale as needed before meals and at bedtime, and furosemide 20 mg daily. Which of these medications is most likely the cause of the muscle pain?
   a. Atorvastatin
   b. Calcitriol
   c. Furosemide
   d. Insulin glargine

115. Ms. Johnson should be taught to monitor bowel function and to avoid constipation because constipation increases risk of:
   a. Hypercalcemia
   b. Hypokalemia
   c. Hyperkalemia
   d. Hyperphosphatemia

116. Ms. Johnson has not responded well to an erythropoiesis-stimulating agent (ESA). Which of the following treatments is indicated specifically for hemodialysis patients with epoetin-resistant anemia?
   a. Iron infusion
   b. L-carnitine
   c. RBC transfusion
   d. Oral ferrous sulfate

117. During hemodialysis, Ms. Johnson, who is lying in the supine position, complains of chest pain, begins coughing, and shows evidence of cyanosis of the distal extremities and lips. To prevent further complications, the nurse should immediately
   a. Clamp the venous line and stop the blood pump.
   b. Provide nasal oxygen at 4 L/min.
   c. Increase the blood flow rate and the dialysate flow rate.
   d. Administer a saline bolus to the patient.

118. In response to these symptoms, Ms. Johnson should be positioned
   a. Upright at 90°
   b. In the semi-Fowler's position
   c. In the Trendelenburg position on the left side, or flat supine
   d. In the Trendelenburg position on the right side

119. Which blood abnormality is a common finding with acute interstitial nephritis?
   a. Decreased hemoglobin
   b. Increased eosinophils
   c. Increased monocytes
   d. Increased lymphocytes

120. How many grams of urea are usually produced and excreted in 24 hours?
   a. 5–10 g
   b. 20–30 g
   c. 40–50 g
   d. 60–70 g

121. The permeability of a dialyzer membrane to water is indicated by its
   a. Transmembrane pressure
   b. Osmotic ultrafiltration
   c. Diffusion pressure
   d. Ultrafiltration coefficient

Refer to the following for questions 122-124:

> Abdul El-Amin is a 56-year-old male who has received a living donor kidney from his 48-year-old brother.

122. Mr. El-Amin received basiliximab perioperatively, and tacrolimus and mycophenolate mofetil (MMF) as immunosuppressive therapy. He was placed on a corticosteroid for 1 week only. Early steroid withdrawal is most associated with which of the following complications?
   a. Hyperlipidemia
   b. Mortality
   c. Acute rejection
   d. Graft loss

123. With kidney transplantation, therapy with basiliximab is primarily used to
   a. Prevent T cell replication and organ rejection.
   b. Potentiate the effects of other immunosuppressive agents.
   c. Reduce the risk of post-operative infection.
   d. Reduce the risk of post-operative renal stenosis.

124. Following hospital discharge a week after a kidney transplantation, Mr. El-Amin had been doing well, but has sudden onset of fever of 38.8 °C, chills, tenderness about the incision, and headache. The urine appears cloudy. The most likely cause is
   a. Acute rejection
   b. Infection
   c. Hyperacute rejection
   d. Delayed graft function

Refer to the following for questions 125-128:

John Bell is a 48-year-old man who has been undergoing hemodialysis for 6 months.

125. Mr. Bell frequently experiences leg cramps during hemodialysis. Which of the following may result in muscle cramping during hemodialysis?

a. Hypervolemia
b. Hypovolemia
c. Low ultrafiltration rate
d. High-sodium dialysis solution

126. Mr. Bell says that he is unable to work or care for his family and is increasingly sedentary because of severe episodes of fatigue. The most important intervention is to

a. Advise a program of exercise.
b. Refer to a social worker.
c. Refer for psychological counseling.
d. Assess for causes of fatigue.

127. When documenting observations about a patient, which of the following is the most appropriate description?

a. "Patient is nervous and upset."
b. "Patient appears to be in a very good mood today."
c. "Patient is sighing and rubbing hands together."
d. "Patient is uncooperative and belligerent."

128. The patient has developed a small aneurysm and asks the nurse to cannulate the aneurysm for the hemodialysis treatment because another patient told Mr. Bell that it would be less painful than cannulation of the fistula. The best response is

a. Agree to cannulate the aneurysm.
b. Tell the patient that there is no reduced pain if cannulating the aneurysm.
c. Advise the patient that cannulating an aneurysm may result in rupture.
d. Tell the patient that the other patient was wrong.

129. The nurse serves as case manager for a patient who lives at considerable distance from the nurse's office in a rural area. The patient uses CAPD and manages fairly well but is anxious about being so far from medical help. The best method of keeping in touch with the patient and managing the patient's care is probably

a. Email
b. Home visits
c. Office visits
d. Video chat

130. A positive Chvostek sign is associated with

a. Hyperkalemia
b. Hypokalemia
c. Hypercalcemia
d. Hypocalcemia

131. When utilizing the "Got Chart" method of contacting a physician by telephone regarding a hemodialysis patient, the first step is to ensure

   a. There are no standing orders that pertain to the situation.
   b. The nurse has checked physician preferences regarding contact.
   c. The nurse has read the most recent progress notes.
   d. The nurse is contacting the correct physician.

132. If a dialyzer is to be reprocessed in 3 hours, the dialyzer must be

   a. Heated to body temperature (37 °C)
   b. Frozen
   c. Maintained at room temperature
   d. Refrigerated

133. Patients are at increased risk of mortality when predialytic albumin levels fall to

   a. <2 g/dL
   b. <3 g/dL
   c. <4 g/dL
   d. <5 g/dL

134. If severe hemolysis occurs during hemodialysis, the patient is most at risk for which electrolyte imbalance?

   a. Hyponatremia
   b. Hypernatremia
   c. Hypokalemia
   d. Hyperkalemia

135. Prior to use of a reprocessed dialyzer, a recirculating rinse with NS should be completed, with recirculating flow rate through the blood compartment and the dialysate compartment of at least

   a. 200 mL/min for BFR and 200 mL/min for DFR
   b. 200 mL/min for BFR and 500 mL/min for DFR
   c. 500 mL/min for BFR and 200 mL/min for DFR
   d. 500 mL/min for BFR and 500 mL/min for DFR

Refer to the following for questions 136-140:

   Andre Robinson is a 76-year-old male with chronic kidney failure. He has begun to gain excessive weight, and blood tests indicate he is no longer adhering to his dietary restrictions.

136. Mr. Robinson admits that he understands his dietary needs but finds cooking too difficult. He has been eating primarily foods delivered from a fast-food restaurant across the street from his apartment. The most useful response is probably to

   a. Refer the patient to a Meals on Wheels program.
   b. Refer the patient to the renal dietitian.
   c. Recommend the patient to an occupational therapist.
   d. Remind the patient of the importance of diet.

137. Mr. Robinson's sister reports that he is having fluctuating periods of inattention, disorientation, and general confusion. Which of the following tools is intended to assess the development of delirium in patients as opposed to other causes of altered mental status?
   a. MMSE
   b. Mini-Cog
   c. Palliative Performance Scale
   d. Confusion Assessment Method

138. The nurse assesses Mr. Robinson's mental status. Which of the following tasks is appropriate to assess a patient's ability to concentrate?
   a. Naming the current president
   b. Providing the patient's social security number
   c. Stating the city and state of residence
   d. Repeating the days of the week backward

139. Mr. Robinson's condition deteriorates, and tests show he has almost reached stage 5 chronic kidney disease, but he is not a candidate for transplantation. His prognosis, even with dialysis, is very poor because of multiple comorbidities. The best solution is to
   a. Carry out a hemodialysis trial.
   b. Discuss prognosis and options with the patient.
   c. Provide palliative care only.
   d. Discuss options with family members.

140. Mr. Robinson's PTH levels are elevated. For a patient with non-dialytic chronic kidney disease and elevated levels of PTH, the KDIGO guidelines recommend treatment with
   a. Vitamin D
   b. Calcium
   c. Prednisone
   d. Cinacalcet

141. The primary difference between glomerular filtrate and plasma is that glomerular filtrate does NOT contain
   a. Amino acids
   b. Glucose
   c. Sodium
   d. Proteins

Refer to the following for questions 142-144:

Alton Whitlow is a 66-year-old male who had a kidney transplantation because of kidney failure associated with diabetes and hypertension.

142. Ten months after kidney transplant, Mr. Whitlow develops severe hypertension and pulmonary edema, as well as increasing signs of acute kidney injury with increasing serum creatinine. The surgeon suspects renal artery stenosis. The test that is most commonly used to confirm the diagnosis is
   a. Angiography
   b. CT scan
   c. MR angiography
   d. Radiograph

143. Which of the following is a risk factor for renal artery stenosis?
   a. Hepatitis B infection
   b. Hepatitis C infection
   c. Cytomegalovirus infection
   d. Fungal infection

144. After confirmation of the advanced renal artery stenosis, the treatment of choice is most often
   a. Vasodilators
   b. Transluminal angioplasty with or without placement of stents
   c. Surgical revascularization
   d. Hemodialysis

145. If imaging shows that the kidneys have atrophied to about one-fifth the normal size, the most likely diagnosis is
   a. Acute glomerulonephritis
   b. Chronic glomerulonephritis
   c. Polycystic kidney disease
   d. Renal cell cancer

146. What is the best time to discuss advance directives with a patient who is diagnosed with kidney failure?
   a. Upon patient request
   b. Early after diagnosis
   c. At stage 4
   d. After initial renal replacement therapy

147. When the nurse instructs a patient on hemodialysis about weight gain, the patient should be advised that the usual goal for interdialytic weight gain is
   a. <0.5 kg/day
   b. <1 kg/day
   c. <1.5 kg/day
   d. <2 kg/day

148. Two patients in the hemodialysis center are afebrile with no complaints at the onset of hemodialysis, but begin to have chills, and each spikes a fever within 45–60 minutes. The most likely cause is
   a. Local infection
   b. A pyrogenic reaction
   c. Dialysis disequilibrium syndrome
   d. Systemic infection

149. A 32-year-old female patient has developed fever, maculopapular rash, pyuria, and acute renal insufficiency, suggestive of acute interstitial nephritis. The most common cause for the development of acute interstitial nephritis is
   a. Hypokalemia
   b. Sjögren syndrome
   c. Systemic lupus erythematosus
   d. Drugs

150. A postmenopausal hemodialysis patient complains of dyspareunia. The most effective treatment is likely
   a. Vaginal lubricant
   b. Sustained-release intravaginal estrogen ring
   c. Psychological counseling
   d. Conjugated estrogen cream

Answer Key and Explanations for Test #2

1. D: Working one-on-one with an experienced nurse is often the best way to improve skills, and can also decrease risks to the patients because being unfamiliar with equipment can lead to errors.

2. A: This is one method of assessing the effectiveness of peritoneal dialysis. This test also helps to identify those with high rate of transport because these patients may rapidly absorb glucose and may need to have shorter dwell times. If the amount of urea and creatinine filtered is inadequate, the patient may need a longer dwell time or more exchanges.

3. A: The reason for eosinophilia in patients with kidney disease is not clear, but there is some indication that eosinophilia is more associated with vascular disease—such as may occur with diabetes—than uremia. Studies have shown that eosinophil counts drop during the first quarter hour of dialysis and then increase markedly at the end of the dialysis session.

4. B: An 18-year-old patient is legally an adult and therefore may choose to discontinue treatment, and there is little recourse if the patient is of sound mind. Because the patient has agreed to stay on medications, the best response is to provide education and support, showing respect for the patient while acknowledging concern. The patient should be thoroughly apprised of signs of uremia, as the patient may change his mind when his condition deteriorates.

5. D: The False Claims Act prohibits any false claims to the United States if the person submitting the claim understands that it is fraudulent. Other actions that are prohibited include billing for goods or services that were unnecessary, billing for services that were provided but were substandard, accepting or giving kickbacks, and unbundling of charges for supplies or services that should be grouped.

6. A: Dialysate usually contains sodium, chloride, and lactate or bicarbonate. Although alternative osmotic agents—such as icodextrin and amino acid solutions—are available, glucose remains the most widely used, although it may result in patients absorbing 200–300 g of glucose daily. This may further result in hyperglycemia and weight gain because of the additional calories, as well as increase the risks of hyperlipidemia and cardiovascular disease.

7. C: Sodium modeling occurs when the sodium level in the dialysate is higher at the beginning of treatment than it is later in the treatment so that the patient's sodium level returns to normal at the end of treatment. The higher the sodium content, the more fluid that is drawn from the tissues into the blood. However, sodium modeling makes some patients thirstier, so that they drink more, and this in turn can result in increased blood pressure.

8. D: The formula for URR is:

$$\left(\frac{[\text{inflow} - \text{outflow}]}{[\text{inflow}]}\right) \times 100 = \left(\frac{[100 - 35]}{100}\right) \times 100 = 65\%$$

URR is used to estimate the amount of urea nitrogen that is removed from the blood by dialysis. The goal is usually about a 65% reduction.

9. A: The nurse should recalculate the target weight loss with the patient to determine which target is correct. Patients should be taught to monitor their own care because anyone can make mistakes, and patients often are very knowledgeable about their conditions and needs.

10. B: One kilogram (2.2 lb) of increased weight represents 1 liter of fluid retention. Dry weight is the optimal post-dialysis weight after excess fluid has been removed. Patients may gain weight because of the glucose in dialysate solutions or lose weight because of lost muscle mass or fat stores, so it is important to reevaluate the patient's dry weight at least every 2 weeks to ensure adequate removal of excess fluids.

11. C: Polycystic kidney disease is an autosomal dominant disorder that usually remains latent until the third or fourth decade of life. It involves both kidneys, with the cortex and medulla filling with multiple large cysts that destroy the kidney tissue.

12. D: This scenario represents one circumstance under which confidentiality can be breached. According to *Tarasoff v. Regents of the University of California*, healthcare workers have a duty to warn individuals who have been threatened by their patient and are in imminent danger. While the police may need to be contacted, the priority in a case of threatened harm against another individual by a patient is to warn that individual. The patient should also be referred to a psychiatrist for evaluation by the attending provider and should be evaluated for uremic encephalopathy, which can result in bizarre behavior, but this is not the priority.

13. D: Urea kinetic modeling is used to monitor the adequacy of dialysis in a measurable way, which allows for necessary modifications to be made as needed, while also providing a data point for trending dialysis efficacy for the patient over time. The "K" represents the dialysis urea clearance rate (measured in mL/min). The "t" refers to the duration of dialysis in minutes. The "V" refers to the estimated volume of fluid in mL in the patient's body as a means to capture the volume in which urea is dispersed throughout the body.

14. D: The next step is to determine the time period for observation, such as a month, quarter, or year. If BSIs are rare, then a longer time period is indicated in order to ensure measurement validity. Then, surveillance criteria and data elements to be collected must be determined, followed by outlining the method for data analysis and methods for data collection.

15. C: Patients should be advised to take the supplement on an empty stomach because taking it with food may decrease absorption. Additionally, patients should avoid enteric-coated preparations and should not take the supplement with phosphate binders. Patients are usually prescribed 325 mg ferrous sulfate three times daily.

16. A: During peritoneal dialysis, the concentration gradient of a substance, such as urea, decreases. That is, more urea diffuses into the instilled dialysate when the concentration is low than when the concentration increases. In order to compensate for this change in concentration gradient, more frequent exchanges can be done (such as is common with APD), or dwell volume may be increased, although this typically cannot exceed 2.5–3.0 L.

17. A: The tunnel extends from the peritoneal cavity through muscle and subcutaneous tissue to the skin. The catheters usually contain a set of cuffs, with one cuff distal to the peritoneum and the other subcutaneously at least 2 cm from the exit with 4 cm being optimal. The cuffs hold the catheter in place, prevent leaks, and provide barriers that reduce the risk of infection.

18. A: The most likely reason is to prevent intradialytic hypotension resulting from inadequate vasoconstriction. Contraindications to this drug include supine hypertension and active cardiac ischemia (although the drug may be administered with coronary artery disease without ischemia). However, if a cooler dialysate solution is being used to prevent intradialytic hypotension, adding midodrine does not provide increased benefit.

19. A: If the patient is not incontinent and is able to use the toilet, then no special precautions are needed. However, healthcare personnel (and others) who are pregnant should avoid the patient for 24 hours after the procedure to avoid exposing the fetus to radiation. The radiation dose is relatively small and is excreted rapidly.

20. A: Glucose in dialysate must be heat-sterilized at low pH in order to decrease generation of glucose degradation products (GDPs), which can irritate the peritoneal membrane. For single-compartment dialysate bags, the dialysate is heated at 5.5 pH because a lower-pH solution would be too painful for instillation. However, in a double-compartment bag, the glucose-containing dialysate is heat-sterilized at about 3.2 pH, while the other compartment is heat-sterilized at an alkaline pH. Then, the two compartments are mixed before instillation.

21. B: Rigid non-cuffed catheters should be used for peritoneal dialysis for a maximum of 3 days, usually only for acute care. These catheters pose an increased risk of infection and should be avoided if possible, but one may be inserted before a chronic cuffed catheter to allow immediate dialysis. Rigid non-cuffed catheters are typically made of a semi-rigid plastic material and may be curved or straight. They are inserted with the use of an internal stylet that facilitates percutaneous insertion.

22. A: With chronic kidney failure, vascular calcification results from hyperphosphatemia, which in turn results in hypocalcemia, because as phosphate levels increase in the serum, calcium levels fall. The decrease in serum calcium stimulates the parathyroid glands to secrete increased PTH. With kidney disease, the body does not respond normally to PTH, so calcium leaves the bones, resulting in osteomalacia, and builds up in the vessels, causing calcification. Additionally, vitamin D, which is needed for the body to properly utilize calcium, is not metabolized normally.

23. D: This patient should not be taking metformin because it may result in lactic acidosis when the serum creatinine reaches this level. Metformin is contraindicated for males with serum creatinine ≥1.5 mg/dL or for females with serum creatinine ≥1.4 mg/dL. Patients with kidney disease who are taking metformin must be closely monitored.

24. A: The goal should be to decrease the patient's low-density lipoprotein (LDL) to (at most) less than 100 mg/dL, although in some cases the goal may be set even lower, such as to below 70 mg/dL. The patient's LDL level is now categorized as borderline high (130–159 mg/dL). Because LDL is the primary cause of atherosclerotic plaques and arterial obstruction, it's important to lower the LDL level and increase the level of high-density lipoprotein (HDL), which functions to remove cholesterol and should be greater than 60 mg/dL.

25. A: Strenuous exercise and red meat may interfere with the results of the test. Serum creatinine indicates the kidneys' abilities to excrete waste. Normal values vary from one laboratory to another but are usually less than 1.2 mg/dL. Elevation of the serum creatinine is an indication of renal disease. Urine creatinine should always be considerably higher than serum creatinine.

26. C: The patient should expect to have a bowel prep the day before the test and to be NPO for 8 hours prior to the procedure. The intravenous pyelogram (IVP) is a fluoroscopic procedure that requires injection of a radiopaque dye and a series of radiographs. Following the IVP, the patient should be encouraged to drink fluids to help flush the dye and should be monitored for signs of allergic response.

27. A: The glomeruli are part of the functioning unit of the kidney, the nephron. The nephron is made of the renal corpuscle and the renal tubule. The filtering unit in the renal corpuscle is the glomerulus (a cluster of blood capillaries) and a sac-like structure that surrounds it, Bowman's capsule. With diabetic nephropathy, the glomeruli become scarred and are no longer able to adequately filter the blood of solutes. The first indication is often the finding of microalbuminuria.

28. D: Antidiuretic hormone (ADH) is released by the pituitary gland in the brain in response to hypovolemia. It increases fluid reabsorption at the renal tubules, decreasing urinary output in an effort to increase blood volume and to increase blood pressure. In addition, as response to hypotension, the kidneys release renin, which converts angiotensinogen (produced by the liver) to angiotensin I, which in turn is converted into angiotensin II by a lung enzyme. Angiotensin II is a vasoconstrictor that helps increase blood pressure.

29. A: This probably represents protein in the urine resulting from changes in the glomeruli that allow proteins to pass into the urine. With proteinuria, patients may also begin to exhibit generalized edema. Changes in urinary patterns are indicative of kidney failure. Patients may also experience more frequent urination and nocturia. The urine may contain blood. Urine may appear more concentrated or less concentrated.

30. B: There may be many reasons that a new team member is less productive than others on the team, including insecurity, lack of knowledge, lack of experience, or poor time management. It often takes new team members time to achieve the same level of expertise as those with more experience on the team.

31. D: Physiologic needs include the need for oxygen, food, elimination, control of temperature, sex, movement, rest, and comfort. The next level of concern is that of safety and security, followed by love and belonging, then self-esteem. Self-actualization is the highest level and is often dependent on meeting needs at the lower levels.

32. B: Patients often express the wish to die, and they have the right to refuse treatment and request no life-saving treatments. However, since the patient did not request a DNR (do-not-resuscitate) order, nursing staff cannot assume that the patient would want no resuscitation efforts made.

33. B: Sediment filters strain residue, such as particles and solutes, from the feed water. The filters are layered, with each layer screening out more and more particles, but the channels in the filter can plug if the sediment builds up, so the water flow through the unit is reversed to flush the sediment out of the filter. This process may be done automatically.

34. C: The FDA publishes *Quality Assurance Guidelines for Hemodialysis Devices* to provide guidance to hemodialysis units and centers and to outline the steps to quality assurance. The FDA has also published a draft guidance for implanted blood access devices, including subcutaneous catheters. Hemodialysis providers must report any problems with the medical devices in use and report all adverse events.

35. C: Urine osmolality indicates the amount of solutes in the urine. If the kidneys are unable to adequately filter the blood and remove waste products, the urine osmolality decreases. While urine osmolality may vary from 250 Osm/kg to 900 Osm/kg, the average adult with normal intake and kidney function has a urine osmolality of 500 Osm/kg to 800 Osm/kg. Therefore, an osmolality of 300 Osm/kg indicates early kidney disease. As urine osmolality decreases, serum osmolality should increase.

36. B: Patients are often confused about discharge plans and anxious about returning home, so a telephone call the day after discharge is often welcome and ensures that the patient understands and follows through with the discharge plan.

37. C: While all the other symptoms (changing patterns of sleep with insomnia, feeling tired and lethargic, and exhibiting psychomotor agitation) are also commonly found with depression, they are also common to uremia and can be mistaken for depression, which does frequently occur with uremia. Repeatedly thinking about dying or imagining committing suicide are always cause for concern.

38. C: UTIs account for 45–47% of infections after transplantation. They impair the function of the donor kidney or lead to loss of the kidney and, in some cases, death. Infection is especially dangerous if it occurs in the first 6 months after transplant. Bacteriuria and UTIs may be asymptomatic because of immunosuppression. Administration of antibiotic prophylaxis and early removal of urethral catheters have helped to reduce infections, but rates remain high.

39. B: Preemptive transplantation is an especially good option if the patient is receiving a donated kidney from a family member or friend, because the surgery can be planned for and scheduled in advance without concern that a kidney may not be available. Another advantage is that long-term costs are decreased; however, the patient must take long-term immunosuppressive drugs.

40. B: The purpose of a "zero lift" program is to prevent injuries, most commonly musculoskeletal disorders involving damage to muscles, nerves, and tendons. While staff can still assist patients to move and ambulate, staff members should avoid manual lifting as much as possible. It is important when instituting a "zero lift" program that staff members are trained in alternate methods, such as the use of assistive devices, and that the necessary equipment is readily available.

41. C: Tricyclic antidepressants are associated with more adverse effects and are usually avoided. Depression adversely affects quality of life and increases the risk of both morbidity and mortality. Depression is common in patients with chronic kidney disease and is often exacerbated by hemodialysis.

42. B: Cognitive behavioral therapy helps patients to change the way they think about things and provides methods to help substitute positive thoughts for negative ones. Patients are taught to recognize automatic thoughts (cognitive distortions) such as all-or-nothing thinking, catastrophizing, "mind reading," and personalization. Treatment is usually relatively short-term (5–20 sessions).

43. C: Resilience is the ability to respond to stressful situations in a healthy and productive manner. A high degree of resilience allows a patient to cope well. Resilience is often associated with a positive outlook, good family support, and spirituality.

44. A: When hemodialysis patients skip treatments and medications, they are putting their lives at risk, and this provides an easy method of suicide. Once patients have decided to commit suicide, they may sometimes appear to be in a better mood, even cheerful.

45. D: The American Kidney Fund provides financial assistance to patients on dialysis through a number of programs:

- Grants Management System (GMS): Patients can apply directly for grants.
- Health Insurance Premium Program (HIPP): Provides assistance with Medicare Part B, Medigap, COBRA, and other insurance premiums.
- Safety Net Grant Program: Assists with treatment-related expenses that are not covered by insurance.
- Prescription drug resources: Provides lists of drug companies with special programs and resources for those without prescription drug coverage.

46. C: Income can influence the patient's access to healthcare, adequate housing, and nutritious foods. Patients with little income often have few of the options available to those with high income. Education may influence the patient's choices and understanding of disease. Occupation may affect the patient's ability to remain employed. For example, blue-collar workers may find it much harder to continue working because of physical limitations when compared to white-collar workers.

47. C: It is also legal to ask if the dog is needed because of a disability, but it is not legal to ask what the disability is, to ask for proof that the animal is certified or trained, or to have the animal demonstrate its skills.

48. D: The primary purpose of using an amino-based dialysate solution for peritoneal dialysis is for nutritional supplementation, as it promotes uptake of amino acids in skeletal muscles. However, the amino-based solution can only be used 1 time daily in order to prevent acidosis and increased serum urea levels. The solution is usually absorbed within 4–6 hours and is most effective if administered after meals to aid in protein synthesis. Amino-acid solution is osmotically comparable to 1.36% glucose.

49. B: The maximal dose of dialysis is 25 mL/kg/hr, as higher rates have not been shown to reduce mortality rates or to improve the rate of recovery. It is important to identify kidney injury as soon as possible and to institute early renal replacement therapy, as any delay increases the risk of death. Use of citrate rather than unfractionated heparin results in better outcomes.

50. C: The best preventive is use of ultrasound for guidance during the procedure. The veins of the neck may exhibit a range of variability, so use of anatomic landmarks may not be sufficient. In some cases, the carotid arteries may also be atypical, increasing the risk of carotid artery punctures and hematoma.

51. C: In order to slow the progression of chronic kidney disease in patients with chronic metabolic acidosis (usually associated with GFR of less than 25 mL/min/1.73 m^2), sodium bicarbonate should be administered to maintain the serum bicarbonate level at 22 mmol/L. It is important to control metabolic acidosis because it also results in increased reabsorption of bone, increasing the risk of fractures. The dose of sodium bicarbonate that is usually administered is 0.5–1.0 mmol/kg/day.

52. C: The patient should be advised to remain ambulatory after instillation and between scans so that intra-abdominal pressure is increased and the tracer enters the pleural cavity. A scan is usually taken immediately on instillation and then at 10-minute intervals (0, 10, 20, 30) for 4 scans. In some cases, another scan may be completed in 2–3 hours.

53. D: The presence of organic material (such as blood or semen) in the urine may give a false positive for a urine albumin dipstick. Other causes of false positives may include alkaline urine, radiocontrast agents, contamination with detergents or disinfectants, and urine specific gravity of greater than 1.030. False negatives are associated with specific gravity of less than 1.010, acidic urine, increased urine sodium, and presence of non-albumin proteinuria.

54. D: Patients who experience intradialytic hypotension are at increased risk of poor outcomes. Blood pressure should generally be maintained at a systolic pressure of at least 90 mmHg. Low predialytic blood pressure is often an indicator for intradialytic hypotension.

55. C: This probably represents poor nutritional status, usually associated with a low serum albumin level. Both poor nutrition and inflammation may result in lowered cholesterol levels. Patients who maintain their serum cholesterol between 200 and 250 mg/dL tend to have a lower risk of mortality, and levels of less than 150 mg/dL are associated with increased risk. There is some debate about the use of statins because of this, but patients on dialysis are also at high risk of cardiovascular disease.

56. D: Up to 70% of patients on dialysis complain of headaches, and dialysis may exacerbate migraines. Headaches may result from hypomagnesemia, although magnesium supplementation must be used with caution in patients with kidney failure. NSAIDs are usually avoided because of their nephrotoxic affects, and aspirin should be avoided with heparin use during dialysis.

57. B: Other causes of the low-pressure alarms include separation of the blood tubing from the venous needle or catheter, decreased blood flow rate, and blockage of the blood tubing before the monitoring site. A high-pressure alarm for venous pressure may indicate blockage of the blood tubing between the venous needle and the monitoring site, infiltration of the venous needle, a poorly functioning central catheter, or access clotting.

58. C: The patient will need to not only take medications but also modify their diet in order to achieve this response. Studies have shown that lowering the HbA1c in adults with chronic kidney disease to less than 6% increases the risk of mortality. If the patient's pre-diabetic baseline HbA1c is available, then the patient's target goal may be individualized to within 10% of normal.

59. C: This procedure requires insertion of a catheter into the bladder and instillation of contrast dye. The dye outlines the bladder contour and shows reflux. The patient is asked to urinate while radiographs are taken; this provides extra information about the patency of the urethra and the bladder tone, as impairment may result in reflux.

60. C: In order to reuse dialyzers, the dialysis center must follow standards developed by the Association for the Advancement of Medical Instrumentation (AAMI). CMS utilizes these standards as well, under their conditions of coverage for ESRD facilities. Standards are set for both manual and automated reprocessing, but most reprocessing is done by companies that specialize in reprocessing because of the cost of equipment and the strict standards. All automated equipment must be approved by the FDA.

61. D: Albumin is the molecule that has the highest molecular weight, calculated in daltons (Da): 66,000 Da. Dialyzer membranes screen for different molecular weights, with the molecular weight cutoff representing the molecule with the highest molecular weight able to pass through the membrane. Larger molecules have greater molecular weight. Creatinine has a molecular weight of 113 Da, urea has a molecular weight of 60 Da, and calcium has a molecular weight of 40 Da.

62. C: Needles should be inserted at least 0.5 inches away from previous needle sites and at least 1.5 inches away from the anastomosis or any sign of stenosis. The arterial needle is placed toward the arterial anastomosis, and the venous needle is placed toward the venous anastomosis (keeping a minimum of 1.5 inches away from the anastomosis). When inserting a needle, the nurse should always consider first where the needle tip will rest.

63. B: About 1 in 10 patients hospitalized for end-stage kidney disease also have a psychiatric disorder, and these conditions may be precipitated or exacerbated by the stress of dealing with a chronic illness, functional and dietary restrictions, and sexual dysfunction. Patients who are on medications for psychiatric disorders may need to have medication protocols modified.

64. D: According to the NHSN Dialysis Event Surveillance guide, the standardized infection ratio (SIR) is calculated based on the number of observed bloodstream infections (BSIs) divided by the number of predicted BSIs, based on national statistics and the number of patients. If the results show an SIR greater than 1.0, then the facility has a rate of BSIs higher than predicted. A score of 1.0

indicates the rate of infection is the same as predicted, and an SIR of less than 1.0 indicates that the BSI rate is lower than predicted.

65. A: Blood tubing for hemodialysis is generally color-coded to help decrease the chance of errors, with arterial tubing color-coded red and venous tubing color-coded blue. Some types of equipment may require custom tubing sets for individual patients. Blood tubing includes patient connectors that connect the blood tubing segments to the patient's needles/catheter ports, dialyzer connectors that allow connection to the dialyzer, and drip chamber or bubble trap to check the arterial or venous pressure. The heparin and saline infusion lines are usually placed on the arterial tubing segment.

66. C: The proper procedure is to place the catheter bag in a container of ice so that the urine remains chilled, and then to collect the urine every hour, placing the collected sample in a refrigerated container until the entire 24-hour collection is completed. The creatinine clearance test usually requires collection for 12–24 hours.

67. B: The recipient cannot be told the donor's location, name, or address. If the recipient wants to contact the donor's family, the recipient can write an anonymous letter that will be forwarded to them. While some recipients have managed to track down a donor family, some donor families may not be receptive, and doing so is a violation of privacy.

68. D: Other antiproliferatives include azathioprine and sirolimus. Mycophenolate mofetil (MMF) inhibits the activation of lymphocytes by preventing their proliferation. Patients must be carefully monitored for adverse effects, which can include infections and malignancies. Nausea and gastrointestinal disturbances are common. Blood tests should be monitored for leukopenia and thrombocytopenia, which can increase the risk of infection and bleeding. MMF is usually administered in oral form.

69. C: Core needle biopsies are usually done under ultrasound guidance. The biopsies can also be done with CT, but CT-guided biopsy is more expensive and exposes the patient to radiation. Core needle biopsies are done with special 18-gauge core biopsy needles. The patient may receive conscious sedation as well as a local anesthetic while in the supine position. The core biopsy is usually obtained from the lower pole of the kidney.

70. A: The initial treatment is usually high doses of corticosteroids to depress the immune system. If the patient does not respond adequately to the steroids, then monoclonal antibodies, such as OKT3 or basiliximab, are administered. In some cases, high doses of an antiproliferative agent, such as mycophenolate mofetil (MMF), may also be administered. Different centers use different protocols, but treatment may be individualized depending on patient response.

71. B: The increased blood pressure, hand tremors, somnolence, and loss of memory are especially indicative of cyclosporine. The cyclosporine level should be evaluated and will probably indicate toxicity. Cyclosporine levels are often taken daily until the optimal dose is established.

72. A: Patients who tend to be hypotensive during hemodialysis should also avoid eating immediately before the treatment. Eating likely causes dilation of the splanchnic venous system and reduces the circulating volume of blood. This effect may continue for up to 2 hours after eating. Oral fluids should also be limited or avoided because it can take up to 10 hours for the fluids to be absorbed into the systemic circulation.

73. C: Placing hemodialysis needles in antegrade position causes less scarring than the retrograde position. When a needle is placed in antegrade position, the blood flows in the direction of the needle, so that the blood flow will hold closed the small flap created by the needle. If the needle is in retrograde position, the needle points in the opposite direction of the blood flow, so when the needle is removed, the blood flow keeps the flap open.

74. D: While general fatigue and weakness may prevent some patients from participating in physical therapy, this patient may benefit from strengthening exercises and a walking or cycling program. The physical therapist can evaluate the patient's physical abilities and determine an appropriate program.

75. A: The use of acupuncture is supported by studies showing that acupuncture provided some relief of symptoms. Both acupuncture and electroacupuncture may provide some relief in the intensity of itching but may not eliminate itching. St. John's wort may react with a variety of different drugs, and its safety for patients on dialysis is not clear.

76. B: Up to 30% of patients on peritoneal dialysis exhibit hypokalemia, although the reasons may vary. Some potassium may be lost in effluent, and patients may have diets with insufficient potassium. Patients usually receive oral potassium supplements as treatment because intraperitoneal administration increases the risk of contamination and peritonitis.

77. D: Pericarditis may occur in up to 10% of patients with uremia. Pericarditis often leads to pericardial effusion as vessels break, leading to cardiac tamponade and—in some cases—cardiac arrest, so rapid intervention to reduce the inflammation associated with uremia is critical.

78. B: In order to achieve this level, the blood flow rate should be set low, to 150–200 mL/min, depending on the size of the individual. The initial hemodialysis session should be limited to 2 hours. These restrictions are important to prevent the development of disequilibrium syndrome, which can occur if blood solutes are removed too quickly.

79. A: The tip of the catheter should extend to the inferior vena cava, as this location improves flow and prevents recirculation. The length required is about 20 cm. While use of the femoral vein is usually discouraged, it does have the advantage of being easy to access without risk of pneumothorax or hemothorax. Although the risk of infection is about the same as for other sites, risks include arterial puncture and retroperitoneal bleeding.

80. C: Ideally, for a patient with chronic kidney disease who will eventually have to have hemodialysis, a phlebotomist should draw blood from the hand veins to avoid trauma to the veins in the arms, which must be preserved for access sites. PICC lines should also be avoided, as they may cause scarring that results in outflow problems. Drawing blood from foot veins should be done only if no other access is available, because of increased risk of complications.

81. D: A patient with chronic kidney disease should have an AV fistula created 6–9 months prior to the expected onset of dialysis because of the prolonged period needed for healing of the AV fistula. Additionally, finding adequate veins may be difficult in patients with chronic inflammation and cardiovascular disease, commonly found in patients with kidney disease. Additionally, an AV fistula may not function properly, so a second AV fistula may need to be created.

82. D: According to the National Kidney Foundation, dialysis should be considered when a patient's eGFR falls to 15. Generally if the eGFR is sustained at 15 or less for three months, dialysis must be started to prevent complications, such as uremia.

83. C: It can be challenging to manage PTH levels and to accurately titrate medications, such as cinacalcet and vitamin D, in order to prevent further complications. If the patient has diabetes, she may already be under the care of an endocrinologist to manage the diabetes. Disease management for the patient with chronic kidney disease often requires multidisciplinary effort.

84. B: Patients with severe kidney disease should avoid MRI with gadolinium contrast agent because it may result in nephrogenic systemic fibrosis, which causes fibrosis of the skin as well as internal organs (similar to scleroderma), and for which there is no treatment. If a patient with kidney disease absolutely must have gadolinium contrast agent because of inability to tolerate other imaging procedures, then the lowest possible dose of gadolinium contrast should be used, and the patient may need to undergo temporary hemodialysis after the MRI to ensure rapid removal of the contrast agent.

85. C: The patient should be advised to limit dietary phosphorus intake to 800–1000 mg/day in order to maintain a normal phosphorus level of 2.5–4.5 mg/dL. Foods and fluids high in phosphorus include chocolate, dark colas, dairy products, organ meats, sardines, oysters, dried beans and peas, nuts, whole grains, bran, and seeds. Patients may be prescribed phosphate binders to absorb some of the phosphorus from foods.

86. D: Some authorities recommend a lower limit of 1500 mg/day in order to keep the serum calcium level in the low to mid-normal range as a means of reducing the risk of vascular calcification. If the patient is taking calcium-based phosphorus binders, this calcium must be added to the dietary intake of calcium. Many foods high in calcium (such as dairy products) are also high in phosphorus and should be avoided.

87. B: In a patient with chronic kidney disease, metabolic acidosis results in increased reabsorption of bone and may also increase the progression of kidney disease. The serum bicarbonate level should be maintained at 22 mmol/L or higher. Treatment to prevent metabolic acidosis is sodium bicarbonate at 0.5–1.0 mmol/kg per day in order to prevent reabsorption of bone. Metabolic acidosis becomes acute when the GFR decreases to about 20 mL/min because the kidneys can no longer filter acids adequately.

88. B: During hemodialysis, usually 100–250 mL of blood is outside of the patient's body at one time. However, if a separation of a bloodline occurs, much more blood may be lost in a small amount of time because the blood flow rate is usually set to pump between 300 and 500 mL per minute. This continuous flow, if undetected, could result in exsanguination. For this reason, it is imperative that the access site be open to view at all times and that the patient be carefully monitored during treatment.

89. C: Change is not necessarily a bad thing, but it may seem threatening to some team members. If the occupational therapist is providing good care, then the nurse must communicate this to team members and help the team to recognize the therapist's contributions.

90. A: The most likely cause is hypersensitivity reaction, usually to dialyzer or blood circuit components. Reactions to dialyzers are most common with new dialyzers ("first-use syndrome") and may range from mild allergic response to anaphylaxis. Although reusable dialyzers are carefully processed and rinsed before reuse, some sterilants, which may cause allergic responses, may remain.

91. C: The usual dose of potassium in dialysate is 2.0 mM, although the dose may be increased to 3.0 mM if the patient experiences hypokalemia. Patients on digitalis also require a dose of 3.0 mM. If this results in higher potassium levels between dialysis treatments, then patients may require routine administration of sodium polystyrene sulfonate resin (Kayexalate). Utilizing potassium doses of 1.0 mM routinely to control hypokalemia is contraindicated because of increased risk of cardiac arrest.

92. C: This probably indicates that the patient has elevated parathyroid hormone, as secondary hyperparathyroidism is common with chronic kidney disease. Cinacalcet is usually indicated when PTH levels increase to 3 times normal range. Treatment, however, puts the patient at risk of hypocalcemia and adynamic bone disease (especially if PTH falls below 100 pg/mL). Calcium and phosphorus levels should be carefully monitored during treatment with cinacalcet.

93. B: With membranous nephropathy, the small vessels and basement membrane of the glomeruli become inflamed and thickened, interfering with the ability of the glomeruli to adequately filter the blood and to reabsorb protein, so that large amounts of protein are excreted in the urine. The goal of treatment is to prevent the progression of kidney damage, but about 1 in 5 patients will progress to end-stage kidney disease over time.

94. D: Iron deficiency occurs in up to 40% of patients with chronic kidney disease and interferes with the action of the ESA. Resistance is defined as no increase in hemoglobin level 1 month after treatment with ESA. Because of the problem of resistance, iron levels should be assessed before beginning ESA treatment. ESA therapy is indicated when hemoglobin levels fall below 10 g/dL.

95. D: The most likely cause is ureteral stenosis, which has caused urine to back up into the kidney. Ureteral stenosis usually occurs relatively late, months or even years after kidney transplant. Causes may vary, including fibrotic changes, an anastomosis that is too tight, or external compression, such as from a lymphocele.

96. B: Although individuals vary greatly, many cultures are more inclined to view illness as caused by an unnatural force, such as a deity or spirit, or as caused by a natural force, such as heat or cold. Patients who consider the source of illness to be outside of themselves may not be receptive to changing personal behavior in order to treat or prevent illness.

97. A: When considering interdisciplinary communication, the nurse's reporting on a patient's condition in a team meeting is an example of collegial communication (i.e., inter-collegial communication). The three basic types of communication are social (chatting about vacation), therapeutic (answering a patient's questions and providing one-on-one instruction), and collegial (communicating with colleagues). Collegial communication may be in spoken form (such as reporting on a patient's condition) or written form (such as writing a summary of the patient's condition or problems).

98. B: The three processes involved in production of urine are:

- Glomerular filtration: This ultrafiltration process produces glomerular filtrate.
- Tubular reabsorption: Much of the filtrate is reabsorbed through diffusion back into the blood, including water, electrolytes, and other solutes. This process demonstrates the ability of the kidneys to concentrate urine.
- Tubular secretion: Potassium and hydrogen ions are secreted back into the urine from the blood to regulate potassium levels and the acid-base balance.

99. B: African American males who are HIV-infected have the most risk of developing HIV-associated nephropathy (HIVAN), although it can occur in all groups, especially in individuals with CD4+ counts of less than 200 cells/mm^3 and a high viral load. Diabetes, hypertension, older age, and co-infection with hepatitis B or hepatitis C are also risk factors. Patients with HIV should have routine kidney function tests, as almost a third of patients will eventually develop some degree of abnormal kidney function.

100. C: Pyelonephritis, an inflammation of the renal pelvis, may affect one or both kidneys and is often the result of an ascending infection, such as cystitis. Chronic pyelonephritis may develop if the patient has longstanding or recurrent urinary tract infections, and this can lead to scarring of the kidneys.

101. B: The purpose of a nitrite production test is to evaluate for the presence of bacteria in the urine, specifically bacteria that produce nitrites, including *Escherichia coli*, *Klebsiella*, *Proteus*, *Pseudomonas*, *Salmonella*, *Citrobacter*, and some species of *Staphylococcus*. A negative finding, however, is not conclusive because negative results may occur when the patient has elevated specific gravity or is taking ascorbic acid. The nitrite production test will not detect the presence of pathogens that are non-nitrite-producing.

102. A: In this situation, the antibiotics are usually taken for 7 days. The duration varies according to the medication prescribed, but first-line antibiotics are usually given for shorter durations (5–7 days) than second-line therapies, such as TMP-SMZ, which is administered for 14 days. The choice of antibiotic should be influenced by resistance patterns in the local area.

103. A: Without a positive frame of mind, the nurse is not likely to convince others that taking action will make a difference. Believing is followed by making a decision to change, and then taking action. Understanding the results of change is usually the last step in the process.

104. C: The usual target is 1.4, to ensure that the patient's level doesn't fall below 1.2. Improving the quality of dialysis may, in some patients, relieve itching to some degree, although the evidence is not clear. Elevated calcium, phosphorus, and parathyroid hormone levels may also cause itching in some patients.

105. B: The intervention most indicated is moisturizers and oil bath, as dry skin is generally the most common cause of itching. High levels of phosphorus, especially, may cause itching. If emollients do not control itching, then antihistamines, such as Benadryl, or other treatments, such as ultraviolet lights or gabapentin, may be considered. Naltrexone or tacrolimus ointment may relieve severe and persistent itching.

106. A: If patients are doing their own cannulations, they should be advised to also don facemasks. Strict aseptic technique and proper hand hygiene with soap and water and/or alcohol-based hand rub are also critical elements in preventing infections. Patients should be advised to monitor staff members for compliance and to insist that staff wear masks and use appropriate techniques.

107. D: Calcium channel blockers may result in cloudy peritoneal fluid for patients on peritoneal dialysis, possibly because the calcium channel blockers result in increased concentration of triglycerides in the solution. While cloudy peritoneal solution is often indicative of infection (cell counts 50–100/mcL), it can also indicate increased levels of monocytes or eosinophils without peritonitis. Peritoneal solution may also become cloudy in the presence of malignancy, blood, or fibrin, and may appear cloudy after an extended dwell period.

108. A: Spiking of dialysis bags places the patient on peritoneal dialysis at high risk for peritonitis because the system can easily be contaminated if aseptic technique is broken. For this reason, closed systems are preferable. The "flush before fill" procedure helps to reduce risk of contamination. Other risk factors include single-cuff catheters and upward-directed exit sites (these should be directed downward or laterally). Hypokalemia also places patients at increased risk of enteric peritonitis.

109. B: The most likely intervention is removal of the catheter and temporary hemodialysis, allowing the peritoneum to rest, along with antifungals as indicated. Once a catheter is colonized, there is little chance that it can be saved. The patient may require hemodialysis for a number of months to ensure that the fungal infection is eradicated before another peritoneal catheter is inserted.

110. C: When patients are undergoing peritoneal dialysis, the most common pathway of infection resulting in peritonitis is intraluminal, usually from poor technique that allows bacteria to enter the system. The most common organisms are coagulase-negative staphylococci or diphtheroids. Other pathways include periluminal from bacteria present on the skin, hematogenous from distant infections, transvaginal from organisms migrating up the uterus and fallopian tubes to the peritoneum, and transmural from organisms migrating from the bowel wall (often associated with colonoscopy or diarrhea states).

111. B: A sample is obtained directly from the peritoneal catheter only in patients who are "day dry" but may have some fluid remaining in the abdomen. Careful aseptic technique must be followed to prevent contamination.

112. C: The sample should be immediately placed into the EDTA-containing tube because a delay of 3–5 hours may result in the inability to identify cell types. Prolonged storage may result in growth of pathogenic organisms. A minimum of 50 mL of fluid should be obtained for the specimen to increase the likelihood of a positive culture.

113. D: Patients undergoing home hemodialysis are required to have a telephone within arm's reach while undergoing dialysis so that they can readily call for help if needed. In some cases, a landline is preferred over a cell phone because it is not dependent on being charged; however, some patients may feel more secure to have both a landline and a cell phone available. The 911 emergency number should be programmed into the telephones for ease of use.

114. A: The medication that is most likely the cause is atorvastatin, as statins are associated with myopathy. The extent of myopathy may vary widely, and symptoms usually recede within 2 months of stopping the medication, although some patients may develop rhabdomyolysis and persistent muscle damage. The patient may tolerate a different statin, or non-statin agents may be used.

115. C: With normal kidney function, only about 5–10% of the potassium load is excreted through the intestines because the kidneys excrete the rest, but with impaired kidney function, the intestines increase excretion up to 25%. Thus, constipation directly impacts potassium excretion, although hyperkalemia usually involves constipation coupled with excessive potassium intake.

116. B: L-carnitine, a naturally produced amino acid, is indicated specifically for hemodialysis patients with epoetin-resistant anemia. Patients on hemodialysis frequently are deficient in L-carnitine because of both poor nutritional intake and loss during dialysis. Patients with low levels of carnitine are more likely to suffer severe anemia that requires treatment with erythropoietin, and are more likely to have epoetin-resistant anemia, so supplementation with L-carnitine may be effective for some patients.

117. A: These symptoms are likely indicative of an air embolism. To prevent further complications, the nurse should immediately clamp the venous line and stop the blood pump to avoid the introduction of more air. Air emboli are usually venous, although arterial emboli can occur.

Hypovolemia and sitting upright during dialysis are risk factors because they reduce venous pressure. Air emboli may result from leaks in the circuit or air in dialysate solution. Air can also be introduced during insertion or removal of central venous catheters.

118. C: In response to these symptoms, the patient should be positioned in the Trendelenburg position on the left side or flat supine (depending on center protocol). Treatment is symptomatic and may include oxygen, intubation and ventilation, and cardiac catheterization or percutaneous needle insertion for aspiration of air from the atrium or ventricle. In some cases, treatment in a hyperbaric oxygen chamber may be utilized to prevent cerebral edema.

119. B: This occurs in about 8 out of 10 patients. While prognosis is usually good, recovery may be a slow process, lasting months. About a third of patients will require temporary acute hemodialysis, although most will not progress to end-stage kidney disease. Identifying and removing the causative agent for drug-induced disease is critical to recovery. In some cases, patients may be treated with corticosteroids if they don't respond to supportive care.

120. B: Urea is formed in the liver from ammonia and is an end product of protein metabolism. If the urine urea value decreases, this means that the kidneys are not adequately filtering out urea, so this can indicate renal disease. Because urea is synthesized in the liver, a decrease can also indicate liver disease. Urea may also be reduced if a patient is on a strict low-protein diet.

121. D: The ultrafiltration coefficient KUF listed for a dialyzer indicates the amount of water that will pass through a membrane at a given pressure in a specified unit of time (generally 1 hour). For example, if the KUF is 10, then 10 mL of water will pass through the membrane for each mL of mercury (mmHg) of transmembrane pressure. So, if the transmembrane pressure were 100, then the patient would lose 1000 mL (10 × 100) of water each hour.

122. C: Early steroid withdrawal (after 1 week) following kidney transplantation is most associated with acute rejection, although steroid withdrawal is not associated with increased graft loss or death. Protocols differ from one center to another. KDIGO guidelines suggest 1 week of steroids and withdrawal or long-term steroids if initially given for longer than a week, but some centers give steroids for 2 weeks or even 3 months and then withdraw them. Early withdrawal of steroids decreases the risk of steroid-associated conditions, such as hyperlipidemia and diabetes.

123. A: With kidney transplantation, therapy with basiliximab is primarily used to prevent T cell replication (which in turn prevents activation of B cells) and organ rejection. It is most often used as an induction therapy, given initially immediately prior to transplantation. Other induction therapies include Thymoglobulin, OKT3, and daclizumab. While induction therapy targets T cells, it also affects other cells and increases the risk of infection, so induction therapy is often given along with antimicrobials to reduce risk.

124. B: The incision should be examined carefully for any drainage or signs of redness. Infections may be superficial or internal, so the patient should be advised to immediately report signs of infection to the physician because immunosuppression increases risk of severe infection.

125. B: Hypovolemia is a primary cause of muscle cramping during hemodialysis. Other common causes include hypotension, high ultrafiltration rate, and low-sodium dialysis solution. Muscle cramps occur when the muscles do not receive adequate perfusion because of vasoconstriction, so cramping frequently occurs with hypotension. Cramping is most likely to occur during the first month a patient receives hemodialysis. Both hypomagnesemia and hypocalcemia may precipitate muscle cramping.

126. D: The most important intervention is to assess for causes of fatigue to determine if treatment may reduce the fatigue and allow the patient to function more normally. Fatigue is a very common effect of chronic kidney disease, occurring in over 60% of patients. Fatigue may be associated with hyperkalemia and anemia.

127. C: This is an objective observation. In documenting, the nurse should avoid subjective descriptions, such as "nervous and upset," "appears to be in a very good mood," and "uncooperative and belligerent," because these descriptions are based on opinion and may be interpreted differently by others. In documenting, the nurse should describe what the patient is actually doing or saying.

128. C: An aneurysm is a weak ballooning area of the vessel, and if it ruptures, the patient could rapidly exsanguinate.

129. D: The best method is probably video chat, such as with Skype or FaceTime. Face-to-face consultation, even per video, is reassuring to a patient who is anxious, and it allows the nurse to see the patient's equipment and monitor the patient's procedures.

130. D: If the patient's facial nerve is tapped at the masseter muscle of the jaw (1 cm inferior to the zygomatic process and 2 cm anterior to the ear), this induces a spasm (tetany) of the facial muscles on the same side because of hyperexcitability of the nerve. Chvostek sign may also be positive with hypomagnesemia and in those with respiratory alkalosis.

131. D: Because of the interdisciplinary care needed by most hemodialysis patients, the first step when utilizing the "Got Chart" method of contacting a physician by telephone is to ensure the nurse is contacting the correct physician (nephrologist, primary care physician, consultant). Before making the call, the nurse should check recent progress notes, standing orders, and physician preferences regarding how, when, and where to call. Additionally, the nurse should determine if the physician needs to be consulted about any other patient, to avoid extra calls. The telephoning nurse should personally assess the patient before calling.

132. D: Dialyzers should be processed within 2 hours. If a dialyzer is to be reprocessed after more than 2 hours (such as in 3 hours), the dialyzer must be refrigerated because the cold helps to retard the growth of bacteria. The dialyzer must be refrigerated during any transportation to another facility for reprocessing. However, the dialyzer should not be frozen. The exact temperature is usually set by the manufacturer and/or the hemodialysis center.

133. C: Patients are at increased risk of mortality when predialytic albumin levels fall to less than 4 g/dL, with increased risk of morbidity with levels less than 3 g/dL. Albumin levels should be monitored before dialysis sessions at least every 3 months because the albumin level is an indicator of a patient's overall nutritional status. If the level is below normal, the cause should be identified and corrected as soon as possible.

134. D: The patient is at risk for hyperkalemia because potassium is released when red blood cells are hemolyzed. Hyperkalemia can lead to cardiac abnormalities and cardiac arrest, so the blood pump should be stopped immediately so that blood with high levels of potassium is not reinfused into the patient. The patient may need treatment for both hyperkalemia and a drop in hematocrit because of the volume of blood that cannot be reinfused.

135. B: A recirculating rinse with normal saline should be completed, with recirculating flow rate through the blood compartment (BFR) of 200 mL/min and recirculating flow rate of 500 mL/min through the dialysate compartment (DFR). The rinse is carried out for a period of 15–30 minutes, being careful to avoid introduction of air into the arterial circuit, as air may interfere with the removal of germicide. Test strips are used to ensure all germicide is cleared from the dialyzer.

136. A: If a patient understands the necessary dietary restrictions, further consultation with a renal dietitian may not be of use. The most useful response is probably to refer the patient to a Meals on Wheels program. Most of these programs provide limited special diets, such as low sodium and/or low carbohydrate, and the choices are likely more nutritious than fast food. Costs are generally low. Many programs deliver a main meal in the middle of the day and include cereal for breakfast the next day and a snack for dinner.

137. D: The Confusion Assessment Method is a tool designed to determine if a patient is experiencing delirium. The 9 factors covered by the tool are the onset, attention level, thinking ability, level of consciousness, orientation, memory, perceptual disturbances, psychomotor abnormalities, and sleep-wake cycle. The tool is intended to be used by those without psychiatric training. Delirium is characterized by fluctuating symptoms. Various factors can trigger delirium, such as electrolyte imbalances and dehydration, putting patients with chronic kidney disease at risk. Delirium may be precipitated by uremic encephalopathy and dialysis disequilibrium.

138. D: Tasks that are appropriate to assess a patient's ability to concentrate are to ask the patient to repeat the days of the week backward, to count backward from 100 by 7s, and to spell the word *world* backward. Patients may also be asked to carry out a simple three-part task (with the directions given one step at a time in case memory is impaired). When assessing intellectual ability and sensorium, the nurse should evaluate orientation, memory, and ability to think abstractly.

139. B: The best solution is to discuss the prognosis and options with the patient so the patient can decide if he wants a trial of hemodialysis or prefers to opt for palliative care only. Family members may be included in the discussion, but if the patient is of sound mind, the decision rests with the patient.

140. A: Hyperparathyroidism, a common finding with kidney disease, acts as a uremic toxin and may result in bone disease. The target PTH level varies with the type of assay used and will increase over time because of resistance to PTH that develops in the bones. After patients are started on dialysis, the target PTH range is usually 2–9 times the normal range.

141. D: The primary difference between glomerular filtrate (the product of glomerular filtration) and plasma is that glomerular filtrate does not contain proteins. Filtrate contains water, amino acids, uric acid, electrolytes, glucose, urea, and creatinine. Plasma proteins are not filtered out of the blood because they are too large to pass through the glomerulus. Glomerular filtration is carried out through the process of ultrafiltration and requires adequate blood pressure as well as blood volume.

142. A: If a patient exhibits signs of renal artery stenosis (refractory hypertension, pulmonary edema, acute kidney injury, bruit over site of transplant), screening procedures may include ultrasound or magnetic resonance (MR) angiography, but confirmation requires angiography. Renal artery stenosis is the one of the most common vascular complications of kidney transplant, with symptoms usually occurring 3–24 months after transplantation. Complications of angiography are not common but can include bleeding at insertion site, perforation of the artery, thrombosis, and arterial dissection.

143. C: Risk factors for development of renal artery stenosis following kidney transplantation include cytomegalovirus infection, surgical trauma, fibromuscular dysplasia, and arterial disease, with atherosclerosis being a primary cause of renal artery stenosis. Other risk factors include the use of a pediatric donor kidney and delay in function of the donated kidney after surgery, as well as lifestyle issues, such as inactivity, obesity, and smoking. One or both renal arteries may be affected. Renal artery stenosis is most common in males over 45 and in females over 55.

144. B: The stenosis may recur in about 1 out of 10 patients, and patients are at risk of acute rejection. If the stenosis is less than 50% and the patient is stable without significant deterioration of kidney function, the patient may be managed conservatively with medications. If angioplasty procedures are unsuccessful, then revascularization may be indicated.

145. B: As the kidneys are damaged, the kidney tissue is replaced with fibrous tissue and the cortex layer of the kidney shrinks to 1–2 mm. The kidney surface becomes very irregular because of scar tissue. While patients may exhibit no symptoms until kidneys are severely damaged, some patients are diagnosed when they develop hypertension and elevated BUN and serum creatinine.

146. B: The best time is early after diagnosis, when the patient is most likely to be able to think clearly and make a considered decision. Advance directives allow the patient to indicate preferences for end-of-life care if the patient is no longer able to do so. In some states, the advance directive may contain a durable power of attorney. However, in some states, the durable power of attorney is a separate legal document that indicates who can make healthcare decisions for the patient if the patient cannot.

147. B: It is common for patients to gain more than this amount. If weight gain is excessive, patients should be cautioned about limiting sodium intake; this restriction is usually more important than fluid restriction, as increased sodium increases thirst.

148. B: Pyrogenic reactions result from pyrogens such as bacterial toxins, and commonly affect more than one patient at the same time. If a pyrogenic reaction is suspected, then the dialysis should be stopped. Whether or not the patient's blood is returned depends on center policy.

149. D: While acute interstitial nephritis may occur as the result of infection or autoimmune disorders, such as Sjögren syndrome or systemic lupus erythematosus, as well as electrolyte imbalances, such as hypokalemia or hypercalcemia, the most common cause is a reaction to drugs (7 out of 10 cases). The drugs that are most often associated with acute interstitial nephritis are cephalosporins, penicillins, sulfonamide-containing diuretics, rifampin, NSAIDs, phenytoin, and proton pump inhibitors. Infections associated with acute interstitial nephritis include cytomegalovirus, histoplasmosis, streptococcal infections, leptospirosis, and Rocky Mountain spotted fever.

150. B: A sustained-release intravaginal estrogen ring has fewer adverse effects than conjugated estrogen cream. The estrogen cream is associated with vaginal bleeding and pain and breast tenderness. Oral estrogen is rarely used with women on hemodialysis. If used, a low dose is needed because the oral estrogen is metabolized more slowly due to the dialysis.

Share Your Story!

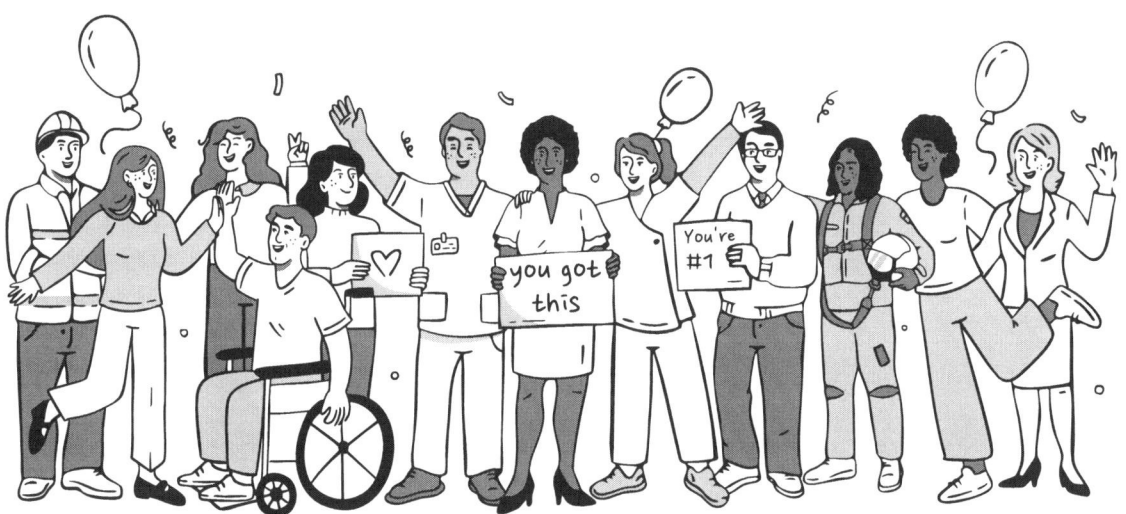

It's Your Moment, Let's Celebrate It!

Share your story @mometrixtestpreparation